Dosage Calculations and Basic Math for Nurses

DeMYSTiFieD

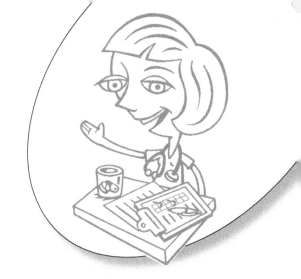

Dosage Calculations and Basic Math for Nurses
DeMYSTiFieD

Jim Keogh, MSN, RN-BC

Second Edition

Mc Graw Hill Education

New York   Chicago   San Francisco   Athens   London   Madrid
Mexico City   Milan   New Delhi   Singapore   Sydney   Toronto

Dosage Calculations and Basic Math for Nurses Demystified, Second Edition

1 2 3 4 5 6 7 8 9 0   DOC/DOC   19 18 17 16 15

ISBN 978-0-07-184968-5
MHID 0-07-184968-8

This book was set in Berling by Cenveo® Publisher Services..
The editors were Andrew Moyer and Cindy Yoo.
The production supervisor was Rick Ruzycka.
Project management was provided by Tanya Punj, Cenveo Publisher Services.
RR Donnelley was printer and binder.

This book is printed on acid-free paper.

Library of Congress Cataloging-in-Publication Data

Keogh, James Edward, 1948-, author.
    Dosage calculations and basic math for nurses demystified / Jim Keogh.—Second edition.
        p. ; cm.
    Includes index.
    Preceded by: Dosage calculations demystified / Jim Keogh. c2009.
    ISBN 978-0-07-184968-5 (pbk. : alk. paper)—ISBN 0-07-184968-8 (pbk. : alk. paper)
    I. Keogh, James Edward, 1948-. Dosage calculations demystified. Preceded by (work): II. Title.
    [DNLM: 1. Drug Dosage Calculations. 2. Drug Prescriptions. 3. Drug Therapy—nursing. QV 748]
    RT68
    615.1′4—dc23
                                                                                              2015000091

This book is dedicated to Anne, Sandy, Joanne, Amber-Leigh Christine, Shawn, Eric, and Amy. Without their help and support, this book couldn't have been written.

—Jim Keogh, MSN, RN-BC

About the Author

Jim Keogh, MSN, RN-BC, is Board Certified in Psychiatric-Mental Health and has written McGraw-Hill's Nursing DeMystified series. These include *Pharmacology DeMystified, Microbiology DeMystified, Medical-Surgical Nursing DeMystified, Medical Billing and Coding DeMystified, Nursing Laboratory and Diagnostic Tests DeMystified, Dosage Calculations DeMystified, Medical Charting DeMystified, Pediatric Nursing DeMystified, Nurse Management DeMystified, Schaum's Outline of ECG Interpretations, Schaum's Outline of Medical Terminology,* and *Schaum's Outline of Emergency Nursing.* His books can be found in leading university libraries including Yale School of Medicine, Yale University, University of Pennsylvania Biomedical Library, Columbia University, Brown University, University of Medicine and Dentistry of New Jersey, Cambridge University, and Oxford University. He is a former member of the faculty at Columbia University and is a member of the faculty of New York University and Saint Peter's University in New Jersey.

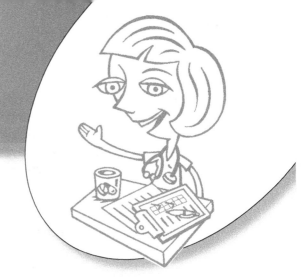

Contents

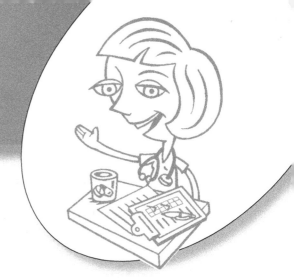

Preface

Calculating the correct dose to administer to the patient is challenging unless you follow a proven approach that is used in *Dosage Calculations Demystified*. Topics are presented in an order in which many nurses and nursing students like to learn them—starting with the basics and then gradually moving on to techniques used in our nation's leading medical facilities everyday to ensure patients receive the proper dose of medication.

Each chapter follows a time-tested formula that first explains techniques in an easy-to-read style and then shows how you can use it in the real-world healthcare environment. You can then test your knowledge at the end of each chapter to be sure that you have mastered nurse management skills. There is little room for you to go adrift.

Chapter 1 Medication Order and Medication

A critical aspect of the nurse's job is to read and understand a medication order and then calculate the dose based on the medication on hand. You might be wondering why you must calculate the dose when the dose is specified in the medication order. The dose in the medication order is the dose of the medicine that the patient is receiving. The calculated dose is the dose of the medicine on hand that is given to the patient to equal the dose in the medication order.

Before learning how to calculate a dose, you'll need to understand how to read a medication order and medication labels, which are covered in this chapter.

Chapter 2 The Formula Method

Based on the medical diagnosis, the physician prescribes a dose of the medication that will improve the patient's condition. Sometimes this is the same dose that appears on the medication label, which means that the patient receives the complete content of the container.

However, the medication might be a different dose and thus requires the nurse to calculate the amount of medication to administer to the patient. Two methods are used to calculate the dose: the formula method and the proportion method. Both methods arrive at the same dose. You'll learn the formula method in this chapter.

Chapter 3 The Ratio-Proportion Method

The goal of the ratio-proportion method is to solve for X using a simple algebraic expression X in the dose. Other elements of the expression are given in the medication order and on the medication label. You'll learn how to use the ratio-proportion method in this chapter and be in the position to choose the ratio-proportion method or the formula method to calculate the dose of medication for your patients.

Chapter 4 Intravenous Calculations

Your patient may require intravenous therapy. How much medication the patient receives depends on the rate of flow of the I.V. The rate is controlled by setting the number of drops of fluid that is administered to the patient each minute. Alternatively, the rate is controlled by the number of milliliters delivered each hour to the patient by a medication pump.

The medication order specifies the medication, the volume, and the time period within which the medication is infused into the patient. You calculate the number of drops or the milliliters setting for the medication pump. You'll learn how to perform these calculations in this chapter.

Chapter 5 Calculating Pediatric Doses

The dose of medication for a pediatric patient must be carefully calculated based on the patient's weight because even a small discrepancy can endanger the youngster's health. Furthermore, there is a limited amount of any medication that the pediatric patient should receive within 24 hours. Before administrating medication, you'll need to determine the total amount of the medication the youngster has already received and then calculate the dose using the patient's weight. You'll learn how to perform both calculations in this chapter.

Chapter 6 Calculating Heparin Dose

Heparin is an anticoagulant (prevents the formation of blood clots) and is administered as a subcutaneous (S.C.) injection or administered in an I.V. and is also used to flush a Hep-Lock that connects I.V. tubing to the patient's vein. So far nearly all dosages that you calculated throughout this book used metric units—milligrams, micrograms, and milliliters. Heparin is different and is measured in USP units (U), which is a standard set by the United States Pharmacopeial Convention Inc. In this chapter you'll learn how to read a medication order for heparin and calculate the proper dose to administer to your patient.

Chapter 7 Calculating Dopamine Dose

Dopamine is a neurotransmitter formed in the brain that affects movement, emotion, and perception. Calculating the proper dose of dopamine to administer to your patient is a little different from the way you calculated the dose of other medications because the prescribed dose is per kilogram and the medication on hand is a concentration. A concentration is a mixture of I.V. fluid that contains a specific amount of dopamine.

Before you calculate the dose for your patient, you must use the prescribed dose to calculate prescribed dose for your patient's weight and you also need to calculate the amount of dopamine in a milliliter of the concentration. You'll learn these calculations in this chapter.

Chapter 8 Calculating Dose for Children Using Body Surface Area

Weight-based dose calculations determine the proper dose based on the patient's weight. Some physicians prefer body surface area rather than weight as the basis for calculating the dose. Body surface area reflects both weight and height and is considered to be the most accurate way to calculate a dose for a child because it considers two measurement of a child. In this chapter you'll learn how to calculate the proper dose of medication for your young patient by using the child's body surface area.

Chapter 9 Enteral Tube Feeding

Patients who have a stroke, tracheoesophageal fistula, esophageal atresia, and other conditions that affect swallowing are a risk for aspiration pneumonia and malnutrition. Physicians take the preemptive strategy of placing the patient on enteral tube feeding (feeding the patient using a tube inserted into the gastrointestinal tract), which greatly reduces the risk for aspiration and assures that nutrients reach the stomach.

Enteral tube feedings usually come in full strength; however, the physician typically orders enteral tube feedings at less than full strength. This requires you to dilute the enteral tube feeding before it is administered to your patient. In this chapter you'll learn how to calculate the fraction or percentage of dilution that must be applied to the full concentration of the enteral tube feeding.

Chapter 10 Positive and Negative Numbers

Positive and negative numbers can be challenging to understand because positive numbers are typically used in everyday calculations. A positive number is a value that is greater than zero. Technically, a plus sign (+) is placed in front of a positive number to indicate that the number is positive; however, it has become common practice not to use the plus sign unless negative number are used. Therefore, no sign in front of the number means the number is a positive number.

A negative number is a value that is less than zero. A minus sign (−) is always placed in front of a negative number to indicate that the number is less than zero. If the minus sign is missing, then the presumption is the value is a positive number.

In this chapter you'll learn how to perform calculations using positive and negative numbers.

Chapter 11 Fractions, Decimals, and Percentage

A fraction is part of a whole of something. For example, each part of a tablet that is split in half is a fraction of the whole tablet. The whole is written as one such as 1 tablet. Each part of the whole is written as less than one as a fraction.

A decimal is a part of a whole of something and another way to write a fraction. A decimal is less than 1 (whole) and more than zero. A decimal value is written by a number that is preceded by a period. The period is called a decimal point. Numbers to the left of the decimal point represents whole things. Numbers to the right of the decimal point represents part of the whole thing.

A percentage is another way of writing a partial value just like using a decimal and a fraction. A percent means per hundred or a value out of a 100 values. This may sound confusing but think of 100 as one whole thing and a value less than a 100 as less than a whole thing.

In this chapter you'll learn how to perform calculations using fractions, decimals, and percentages.

Chapter 12 Ratios and Proportions

A ratio is a mathematical expression for a written statement that compares two things. The expression defines how these things compare to each other. A comparisons commonly written in a healthcare facility is the number of nurses to care for a specific number of patients

Think of proportions as a recipe for making a cake. A cake has ingredients, the amount of each is clearly defined in the recipe. The relationships of ingredients are specified as a ratio. If you want to make a 12-inch cake, then use the ratio of ingredients specified in the recipe. But what if you want make an 18-inch cake? You need to proportional increase the amount of ingredients based on the ratio of ingredients.

In this chapter you'll learn how to perform calculations using ratios and proportions.

Chapter 13 Equations

An equation is an expression of equality using numbers, symbols, and mathematical operations. At first the concept of an equation may seem challenging to understand; however, let's explore this concept in plain English. You can say that: Bob is of the same age as Mary. This is an equation because you are saying that Bob and Mary are of the same age. You can write this as a mathematical equation as: Bob's Age = Mary's Age. In this example, the equal sign (=) is referred to as the equivalent operator. Values on both the left side and the right side of the equal sign are the same value.

In this chapter you'll learn how to create and solve equations.

Final Exam—Parts 1, 2, and 3

Test your skills by taking all three parts of the final exam.

Appendix A Answering Tricky Questions

All dose calculation questions that you'll be asked on a test can be solved using formulas learned in this book or by using basic math that you learned in grammar school. However, some questions are purposely written to confuse you. In this chapter, you'll see tricky questions that are similar to those that you find on tests and you'll learn ways of solving those questions.

Appendix B Quick Reference

Right before a test you probably want to refresh what you've learned through this book. The "Quick Reference" is the only place you need to look. There you'll find a summary of all the formulas and other key information needed to pass your dose calculation test.

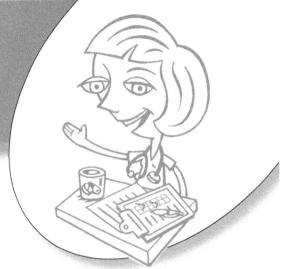

Part I

Dosage Calculations

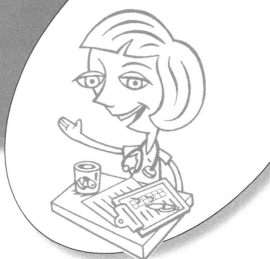

chapter **1**

Medication Order
and Medication

KEY TERMS

Documenting Time	Medication Order Renewal
Expiration Date	Parts of a Medication Order
How to Take Off an Order	PRN Medication Order
Medication Labels	Strength of the Medication

Before any medication is administered to a patient, the nurse must read and understand the medication order and then calculate the dose based on the medication on hand. You might be wondering why you must calculate the dose when the dose is specified in the medication order. The dose in the medication order is the dose of the medicine that the practitioner wants to administer to the patient for providing a therapeutic effect.

Sometimes the dose ordered by the practitioner is the same as the dose contained in the medication package. This is referred to as a **unit dose package**. There is no need to calculate the dose because the medication package contains the exact dose ordered by the practitioner.

Other times the dose in the medication package differs from the medication dose ordered by the practitioner. That is, the medication package may have less than or more than the dose referred to as a **multidose package**. The nurse must calculate the correct dose of the medication to administer to the patient. Sounds confusing? This will be crystal clear after you finish the next chapter.

However, you'll need to understand how to read a medication order and medication labels before learning how to calculate a dose.

1. Medication Order

A patient has aches, pains, and other symptoms (subjective) and goes to a practitioner to relieve those symptoms. The practitioner assesses the patient for objective data called **signs** that lead to a medical diagnosis and treatment plan.

For example, the patient complains about a sore throat (**symptom**). Upon examination, the practitioner notices red and swollen tonsils, white patches on the patient's throat, swollen lymph glands in the neck, and a temperature of 101°F (signs) that might lead to the medical diagnosis of strep throat.

Medication is prescribed as part of the treatment plan for many medical diagnoses. The prescription is a **medication order** that is sometimes referred to as a physician's order. Today medication orders are typically electronically written using a **computerized practitioner order entry** (CPOE) system.

Medication orders can be written on paper in urgent situations when there is no time to enter the order into the CPOE system. The practitioner may give a verbal medication order to a registered nurse (RN) such as in the emergency department. The practitioner might also telephone a medication order to the nurse or pharmacist if the practitioner is not on premises and the patient requires the medication immediately. The practitioner must sign the order within 24 hours depending on the health care facility's policy.

Medication orders are transcribed from the medication order to the patient's medication administration record (MAR). The MAR is a schedule for administering medication to the patient and documenting when and by whom the medication was administered.

Many health care facilities use an electronic medication administration record (eMAR). CPOE medication orders are automatically transmitted to the pharmacy. A pharmacist electronically transcribes the medication order to the eMAR. This is referred to as **taking off the order**. The nurse then reviews and verifies medication orders on the eMAR in a process called **cosigning** the transcription of the order to the eMAR.

Some health care facilities use a paper MAR. Medication orders are transcribed by hand to the paper MAR by a nurse. Another nurse reviews and verifies the transcriptions and initializes the entry into the MAR.

Parts of a Medication Order

There are seven parts of a medication order. If any part is missing, then the medication order is incomplete and the medication cannot be administered to the patient. The practitioner must be immediately informed of the situation and the medication order must be corrected.

The nurse is exposed to legal and administrative consequences if the nurse administers medication based on an incomplete medical order even if the nurse knows the information that the practitioner intended to write in the medical order.

Let's say that the practitioner prescribed CIPRO (Bayer AG) for a urinary tract infection but forgot to include the dose in the medical order. The nurse has worked with the practitioner for years and knows that the practitioner routinely prescribed 250 mg of CIPRO every 12 hours for urinary tract infections. Furthermore, this is the recommended dose by the hospital's pharmacy. The nurse cannot administer CIPRO because the dose is missing from the medical order.

Patient Identification

The patient must be clearly identified on the medication order to prevent the medication from being administered to the wrong patient. The patient is identified by patient's number, patient's full name, and date of birth. This information must be identical to the information on the patient's wrist band. Furthermore, the patient must tell the nurse verbally his or her name and date of birth to confirm the identity.

NURSING ALERT

A patient's name by itself can be misleading because there could be two patients in the same unit having the same full name. A patient's name combined with the patient's date of birth is a preferred method of identifying the patient. The patient's medical record number and visit number are secondary patient identifiers.

Date and Time of the Medication Order

Each medication order must specify the month, day, year, and time that the practitioner wrote the medication order, which is referred to as the **time stamp**. Do not confuse the time stamp of the order with the time to administer the medication. The medication order will specify when to administer the medication.

Depending on the medication, some health care institutions have a policy that specifies when a medical order expires. This is commonly called a **cutoff time** and is used frequently for antibiotics. The date and time of the medical order is used to determine when this time period begins.

Furthermore, a practitioner might want the medication administered for a specific number of days that begins from when the medication order is written.

Medication Name

The practitioner must clearly write either the brand name or generic drug on the medication order. A **brand name drug** is a medication protected by a patent usually held by a company that discovered, tested, and received approval from the Food and Drug Administration (FDA) to sell the drug.

After the patent expires, other pharmaceutical companies can manufacture a bioequivalent medication referred to as a **generic drug. Bioequivalent** means that the generic is in identical dose, strength, route of administration as the brand name medication. For example, CIPRO is the brand name of a synthetic antibiotic sold by Bayer AG, the generic name being ciprofloxacin.

> ### NURSING ALERT
>
> Brand names are printed in all capital letters. Generic names are in lowercase letters and in a different typical face.

Call the practitioner to clarify the medication order if the medication name is illegible. Never try interpreting a practitioner's handwriting because your misinterpretation can have tragic results. There are medications that have very similar names, such as CELEBREX and CEREBYZ. CELEBREX is used to treat pain and reduce inflammation while CEREBYZ is used to control seizures.

Medication Dose

The medication dose specifies the strength of the medication and is the amount of the medication that the patient is to receive. The dose in the medication order includes a value followed by a unit of measurement such as 250 milligrams, which is abbreviated as mg.

Errors can occur when abbreviations are used for the unit of measurement because the abbreviation can be misread as part of the value. For example, U was used as the abbreviation for units, which is the measurement used for insulin. A practitioner could write the following as the dose (see Figure 1–1).

The handwritten U is poorly written. However, the error is easily detected by the nurse because if the value of the dose is 20, as it can be interpreted, then the medication order is missing the unit of measurement for the value and therefore isn't a valid medication order.

A similar problem occurs with the abbreviation for international units, which is IU. A poorly written U can be misread as a V resulting the abbreviation being read as IV instead of IU. This too can be caught because the medication order would be missing the unit of measurement.

The **Joint Commission on Accreditation of Healthcare Organizations (JCAHO)** developed a list of abbreviations that should not be used, which are illustrated in Table 1–1. Some health care facilities have policies that add to this

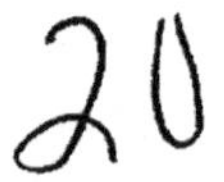

$$20$$

FIGURE 1–1 • Looks like a 20 but really is 2 U.

do-not-use list of abbreviations and instead require practitioners to write out the complete word.

Another common error occurs with decimal values. It is easy to miss the decimal point. For example, .2 mg could be misread as 2 mg or 5.0 mg can be misinterpreted as 50 mg. Practitioner must use a leading zero for decimal values such as 0.2 mg and drop values and exclude the decimal point and zero if no decimal value is used such as 5 mg.

> **NURSING ALERT**
>
> Many health care facilities use CPOE systems to capture medication orders electronically greatly reducing the likelihood that the order will be misinterpreted by the nurse.

Medication Route

The practitioner must specify the way the medication is to be administered to the patient, which is referred to as the *route*. The route is typically identified by the common abbreviations given in Table 1–2.

TABLE 1–1 Do Not Use Abbreviations

Do Not Use	Use in Place	Problem
U	Unit	Misread for zero
IV	International Units	Misread for IV for 10
Q.D., QD, q.d., qd	Daily	Confusing to read
Q.O.D., QOD, q.o.d., qod	Every other day	Confusing to read
.X mg	0.X mg	Decimal point overlooked
X.0 mg	X mg	Decimal point overlooked
MS	Morphine sulfate	Can be confused with magnesium sulfate
MSO_4	Morphine sulfate	Can be confused with magnesium sulfate ($MgSO_4$)
$MgSO_4$	Magnesium sulfate	Can be confused with morphine sulfate (MSO_4)

TABLE 1-2 Abbreviations for Medication Administration Routes	
Abbreviation	**Route**
P.O.	By mouth
I.D.	Intradermal
I.M.	Intramuscular
I.V.	Intravenous
S.C.	Subcutaneous
T.D.	Transdermal

Medication Administration Time and Frequency

The practitioner prescribes the time and frequency of drug administration based on a number of factors including absorption, side effects, interactions with other medication, and the desired effect of the drug on the patient.

The time when the medication is given to the patient is usually at fixed hours according to the health care facilities policy such as 6 PM meds. Sometimes practitioners will prescribe a specific time to administer the medication, but many times the practitioner specifies the frequency. The eMAR system automatically determines times to administer the medication based on the health care facility's policy if the practitioner uses CPOE. The nurse determines the medication administration time based on the health care facility's policy if a paper MAR is in use.

Table 1–3 contains abbreviations that are used to specify the frequency of when to administer medication.

Signature

Every medication order must be signed by the practitioner. CPOE medication orders are electronically signed by the practitioner based on the practitioner's log on identification. Written order must have the practitioner's signature. The signature must be legible on the medication order otherwise the medication order is invalid.

NURSING ALERT

Practitioners who are in training typically require a senior practitioner to cosign medication orders, depending on the health care facility's policy.

TABLE 1–3 Frequencies of Administering Medication and Abbreviations

Abbreviation	Frequency
$\bar{a}$	Before
a.c.	Before meals
b.i.d. or bid	Twice a day
b.i.w.	Twice a week
h or hr	Hour
h.s.	Hour of sleep or at bedtime
min	Minute
noc or noct	At night
o.n.	Every night
$\bar{p}$	After
p.c.	After meals
q.	Every or each
q.a.m.	Every morning
q.h. or qh	Every hour
qXh	Every X hour where X is the number of hours
qhs or q.h.s.	Every night at bedtime
q.i.d. or qid	Four times a day
Stat or STAT	Immediately or at once
t.i.d. or tid	Three times a day
t.i.w.	Three times a week
PRN	As needed

PRN Medication Order

A **PRN medication order** directs the nurse to administer the medication as needed by the patient based on criteria established by the practitioner. The criteria are referred to as **parameters**, such as range of blood pressure, a range of temperature, or a range of pain.

The practitioner must specify the patient identity, date and time of the medication order, name of the medication, dose, and route, parameters, and sign the order. Without any of these, the medication order is invalid.

Medication Order Renewal

Although, the practitioner determines when to discontinue a medication order based on the patient's condition, health care facilities have a **medication order**

renewal policy that requires certain medication orders automatically discontinued after a specified period of time. The practitioner must write a new medication order if the medication is to be continued.

A common practice is to have all medication orders discontinued after 14 days. There are exceptions, which are shown in Table 1–4.

2. The Medication Administration Record (MAR)

The MAR is used to schedule when patients are to receive medication and record when the medication is administered and who administered it. Many health care facilities use an eMAR. Although the form differs among health care facilities, each has the same information.

- **Patient Information**: This includes the patient's name, identification number, room number, diagnosis, and allergies.
- **Schedule Medications**: These are medications that are given regularly to the patient to maintain a therapeutic level such as once a day for seven days.

TABLE 1–4 Examples of When Medication Orders Are Automatically Discontinued

Medication	Discontinued
PRN-controlled medication	72 hours
Anticoagulants	24 hours
	14 days, if the physician specifies the duration of the treatment
Antibiotics	10 days
Antineoplastic	24 hours
	7 days, if the physician specifies the duration of the treatment
Parenteral nutrition	4 days
Schedule II medication (high potential for abuse)	72 hours
	7 days, if the physician specifies the duration of the treatment
Schedule III (moderate physical dependency)	7 days
Schedule IV (limited physical dependency)	7 days
Schedule V (log potential for abuse)	7 days

- **Single Orders**: These are medications that are administered once for an immediate effect such as epinephrine given STAT for anaphylactic shock.
- **PRN Medications**: These are medications given as needed such as non-steroidal anti-inflammatory drug for pain relief.
- **Signature**: The name of each nurse who administers medication to the patient is identified by the nurse's name, which corresponds to the nurse's ID and password that is used to log onto the eMAR.

Pharmacies in many health care facilities distribute medication in unit dose packages, where the complete dose for the patient is contained in one package, where possible. For example, folic acid (see Figure 1–2) is distributed in one 1 mg tablet per package. This reduces the chance that the nurse may give the patient too much medication (higher dose) or too little medication (lower dose).

The eMAR typically indicates the number of packages that make up the full dose below the medication name. Figure 1–2 shows [1 × 1 mg per dose]. This means one package contain a 1-mg dose. This helps the nurse identify the number of medication package required to administer the medication to the patient.

Health care facilities that have yet to convert to eMAR use a paper MAR. The paper MAR contains the same information as the eMAR except that the nurse must initial each time the medication is administered using a pen (Figure 1–3). There is a signature section at the bottom of the paper MAR for the nurse to initial and sign. Anyone reading the MAR can match the initial of the nurse who administered the medication to the initial and signature in the signature section of the MAR to learn the name of the nurse who administered the medication.

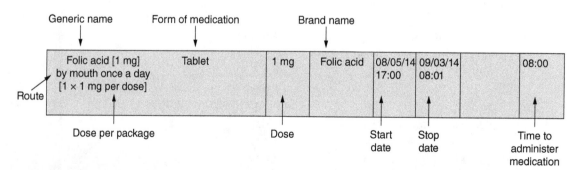

FIGURE 1–2 • Shows a typical eMAR entry that includes both the generic and brand names of the medication, route, form of the medication, dose, start and stop date, and the time to administer the medication.

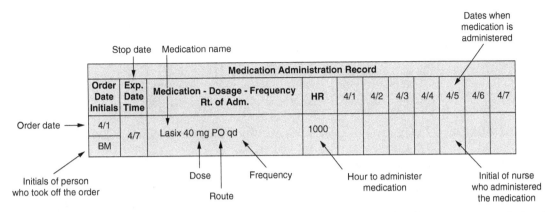

FIGURE 1–3 • The paper MAR requires the same information as the eMAR except that the nurse must enter by hand when the medication was administered to the patient.

> **NURSING ALERT**
>
> A paper MAR is used to administer medication to patients when the eMAR is unavailable such as during a power failure.

3. Creating a New MAR

The practitioner assesses the patient during the admission process to explore problems reported by the patient. The practitioner may order medical tests to gather information about the patient's condition. After receiving test results, the practitioner reaches medical diagnosis and then orders a course of treatment to address the patient's problem, which typically includes writing medication orders.

Medication orders are typically written by the practitioner using a CPOE system. The CPOE system enables the practitioner to write medication orders—as well as nonmedication orders—by first selecting the patient and then entering the name of the medication. The CPOE system displays all the dosage and routes available from the health care facility's pharmacy. For example, Figure 1–4 shows the available dosages for Motrin. The practitioner selects the desired dosage and route and then submits the order. The CPOE system uses the practitioner's ID and password as the electronic signature for the order.

Medication orders are electronically transmitted to the health care facility's pharmacy. A pharmacist reviews the order before electronically transcribing **(taking off the order)** the order onto the eMAR. The eMAR is then electronically made available to nurses who are responsible for medicating the patient.

	Description
Save	Motrin 200 mg orally once
Save	Motrin 800 mg orally 3 times per day
Save	Motrin 800 mg orally once

FIGURE 1-4 • The CPOE system presents the practitioner with available dosages for Motrin.

Before the medication can be administered, the nurse my also verify that the pharmacist properly transcribed the order using a process called **cosigning**. The nurse compares elements of the order to the corresponding entry in the eMAR.

If elements of the order match the eMAR entry, then the nurse electronically marks the eMAR entry as verified (Figure 1–5). If there is a mismatch, the nurse marks the eMAR entry as inactive and then contacts the pharmacist and the practitioner for clarification. Only medication entries marked as verified can be administered to the patient.

NURSING ALERT

Nurses are obligated to temporarily inactive an eMAR entry if there is a question of patient safety. This is sometimes referred to as a nurse hold. The nurse then contacts the practitioner for clarification. The practitioner then decides whether or not the medication is to be administered or the order modified or discontinued.

01 ☒ 07/11/2014 08:00   **Stop:** 08/09/2014 08:01   **Nurse Ordered:** ☐
Ordering Dr:
Rx Entered By: **Schedule**
Pharmacy Verified by: | 07/11/2014 08:00 | Fri |
Pharmacy Verified: 07/11/2014 06:19 | 07/12/2014 08:00 | Sat |
Entered Date Time: 07/11/2014 06:19 | 07/13/2014 08:00 | Sun |
Route: BY MOUTH
Frequency: DAILY
                    ONCE A DAY
Infuse Over:
Rate:
Drug: DIGOXIN (LANOXIN)
Dose: 125 MCG
Strength: 125 MCG
Status: ⦿ Verified ◯ Inactive

FIGURE 1-5 • The nurse compares elements of the medication order to the entry in the eMAR and either verifies or inactivates the entry depending if the entry matches the order.

The MAR is created by hand using a printed MAR in health care facilities who have not adopted an electronic medication administration system. When a patient is admitted to the health care facility, the practitioner write initial medication orders that are transcribed by the pharmacist on to a printed MAR. The printed MAR is printed at the nurse's station and then placed in a loose leaf binder (the MAR). The nurse initials the appropriate place in the MAR each time the nurse administered medication.

Printed MARs are typically printed once a week. The nurse transcribes by hand medication orders that are issued between printings. Transcribed orders must be cosigned by another nurse before medication can be administered to the patient.

After each print of the MAR, the nurse compares the previously printed MAR and the hand written transcriptions to the newly printed MAR before the newly printed MAR is used to administer medication.

4. Information About Medication

The MAR is a time-saving tool because it contains information needed to administer medications to a patient, except for orders that are cancelled or have not been taken off as yet. It is for this reason that you must always review the latest medical orders before administering any medication.

For each medication, the MAR contains the following:

- **Order Date**: This is the date that the practitioner ordered the medication.
- **Expiration Date**: The order is no longer valid on or after the expiration date.
- **Medication Name**: This is usually the brand name of the medication.
- **Dose**: The amount of the medication the patient receives.
- **Frequency**: The number of doses the patient receives.
- **Route of Administration**: The route in which the medication is given to the patient.
- **Site of Administration**: Where was the medication administered if medication was administered in an injection?
- **Date and Time**: The day and hour that the medication must be administered.

5. Using the MAR

At the beginning of each shift, the primary nurse for a patient reviews the MAR and identifies medications scheduled to be administered to the patient during the shift. The **primary nurse** is the nurse who is assigned to care for the patient during the shift. The primary nurse also reviews the patient's chart for any new orders or cancelled orders that were written since the MAR was last updated. These orders if they exist are then taken off by the primary nurse, if the paper MAR is used, or verified if the eMAR is used.

> ### NURSING ALERT
>
> Make a note of orders that are scheduled to expire at the end of the shift. Depending on the patient's condition and the nature of the order, you may want to ask the practitioner if the order should be renewed.

Next, each medication is located on the unit. Medications delivered regularly by the pharmacy are usually placed in the patient's drawer in the medical cabinet or in the medication room. Each is labeled with the patient's name, identification, and room number. It is important to locate medications at the beginning of the shift, thus allowing time to follow-up with the pharmacy if the medication cannot be found.

Some health care facilities use an electronic medication dispensing device such as a *Pyxis, manufactured by CareFusion Corporation*, or *Acudose, manufactured by McKesson Corporation*. The nurse removes medication from the medication dispensing device before administering the medication to the patient. The medication dispensing device keeps an ongoing tally of the medication on hand and medication dispensed.

Before preparing to administer medication, one last check is made of the medical order to determine if the practitioner cancelled the order or prescribed new medication. This is an important step since in a busy unit; the primary nurse may not have the opportunity to speak directly with the physician.

The eMAR application is typically accessible on a computer located on a mobile cart referred to as a **computer on wheels (COW)**. Depending on the health care facility, the COW is either wheeled to the doorway of the room or wheeled to the patient's bedside depending if the COW has a tethered or wireless scanner. A tethered scanner is a handheld bar code reading device that is wired to the COW and used to scan the bar code on the patient's wrist band

and medication packages. A wireless scanner is a handled bar code reading device that uses Wi-Fi rather than a wire to transmit bar code information to the computer.

The scanner is used to scan the patient wrist band, which confirms that the nurse is going to administer the medication to the right patient. Each medication is then scanned ensuring that the correct medication is being administered.

> **NURSING ALERT**
>
> The nurse must ask the patient for the patient's name and date of birth and not rely solely on the wrist band bar code to identify the patient.

Paper MARs may or may not be taken to the patient's room when administering medication depending on the policy of the health care facility. The MAR must be updated immediately after administering the medication. Other health care facilities require the primary nurse to update the MAR immediately upon returning to the nurse's station after administering the medication to the patient. This leaves room for error since the primary nurse can easily be distracted and fail to remember to update the MAR.

> **NURSING ALERT**
>
> Document in the paper MAR after—not before—you administer medication.

6. Taking Off Orders

When using a paper MAR, medication orders must be copied to the MAR. This process is called taking off order. This is a critical process because failure to accurately transfer the order can have serious consequences for the patient.

Many health care facilities require a RN to take off orders; however, some health care facilities authorize trained staff such as a unit secretary to take off orders if reviewed and signed off by a RN.

Orders for medication contain most but not all the information that must be entered into a MAR. Practitioners typically don't specify the exact time to administer scheduled medication. Instead, practitioners use medical abbreviations to indicate the number of doses to administer to the patient.

The primary nurse is responsible for translating this into a medication schedule when taking off the order using the health care facility's policy as a guide. Some health care facilities require that medication ordered for once a day be given at 10 AM.

How to Take Off an Order

Let's say that the practitioner wrote the following prescription:

Lasix 40 mg P.O. every day

This medication is considered a scheduled medication because the order indicates that the patient will take this medication every day until the order expiration date—generally 30 days after the initial order is written depending on the medication.

In an eMAR system, the pharmacist takes off the order.

In a paper MAR system, the practitioner writes the order on paper and places the order in the patient's chart, then flags the chart. **Flagging the chart** is a signal that there is a new order written for the patient. The flag might be a color coded dial on the spine of the chart or extending the paper order beyond the top of the chart and placing the chart on its side on the chart rack.

The flag alerts the primary nurse that there is a new order written for the patient. The primary nurse then takes off the order onto the MAR. A copy is sent to pharmacy and the pharmacist will verify the order, fill it, and send the medication back to the unit. The pharmacy will then ensure that the medication order appears on the next printed MAR.

PRN Orders

A PRN medication is medication that the primary nurse may administer to the patient if the patient experiences specific signs or symptoms. The specific sign or symptoms is called a **parameter** and entered as part of the order. The primary nurse must assess the patients and determine that the patient shows the sign or symptom specified in the PRN medication order before the primary nurse can administer the medication to the patient.

Figure 1–6 shows a PRN order for TYLENOL that states that the nurse can administer 650 mg of TYLENOL every 6 hours as needed if the patient has pain greater than four or a temperature greater than 101°F. The primary nurse cannot administer TYLENOL unless these symptoms exist.

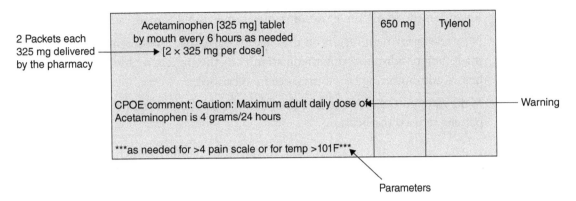

FIGURE 1-6 • Pain and temperature parameters in the medication order specifies when the primary nurse can administer the medication.

7. Avoid Common Errors When Using the MAR

Errors can occur when taking off orders and recording when medication is administered to a patient resulting in over- or undermedicating the patient or administering incorrect medication.

Steps can be taken to ensure that the most common of these errors are avoided.

Here's what you need to do:

- Use abbreviations that are approved by The Joint Commission and adopted by your health care facility. For example, all health care facilities require that "daily" replace the abbreviation OD and "every other day" be used in place of QOD. Always write the full word if you are unsure of the abbreviation to write. Refer to your facilities' Dangerous Abbreviations policy for clarification.

- Avoid confusion writing numbers by dropping the zero following a decimal if the dose is a whole number and use a zero to the left of the decimal if the dose is a fraction. This is a The Joint Commission requirement. Write 1 mg instead of 1.0 mg and 0.5 mg instead of .5 mg.

- Be sure that your full name, title, and initials appear on the paper MAR before initializing that you administered medication.

- Update the MAR immediately after you administer medication to a patient.

- Write legibly on all documents. Assume no one else can read your handwriting so make whatever you can easy to read.

- Record in the MAR the reason for administering PRN medication.
- Note the assessment results on the MAR if particular assessments must be made before administering medication (i.e., the patient's blood pressure before administering blood pressure medication).
- Make note on the MAR or in a progress note in the patient's chart why a patient refused medication.

Documenting Time

Ten o'clock meds are given at what time? This sounds like a joke, but it points to a real problem that occurs in health care facilities. There are two 10 o'clocks in a day—morning and evening.

There are two ways in which the time of the day can be specified:

- Use the AM (**ante meridiem**) and PM (**post meridiem**).
- Use **military time**.

Many health care facilities use military time to avoid any misinterpretation of the time. Military time uses a 24-hour clock that begins with 0000 and ends with 2400. The first hour of the day is 0100, which is 1 AM. Noon time is 1200. Instead of starting over with 1 PM, you continue with the sequence. 1 PM is 1300. Midnight is 2400.

Converting From Traditional Time to Military Time

Military time is confusing because the first 12 hours of the day is basically the same as using AM; however, military time becomes tricky after noon because different numbers are used to indicate the time.

You could count by adding 1 to 12 (noon time) or use these conversion tips.

For AM

1. Remove the colon between hours and minutes.
2. Insert a leading zero if the number is less than 10.

For PM

1. Remove the colon between hours and minutes.
2. Add 1200 to the time.

For example, converting 9:30 AM to military time,

A. 930

B. 0930

Converting 2:30 PM to military time,

1. 230

2. 230 + 1200 = 1430

Converting Military Time to Traditional Time

Determine traditional time from military time is straightforward. Here's what you need to do:

If the military time is greater than 1200

1. Subtract 1200 from the time.

2. Insert the colon between the hours and minutes.

3. Insert PM at the end of the time.

If the military time is less than 1300

1. Drop the leading zero, if there is one.

2. Insert the colon between the hours and minutes.

3. Insert AM at the end of the time.

For example, converting 1430

1. 1430 − 1200 = 230

2. 2:30 PM

For example, converting 0930

1. 930

2. 9:30

3. 9:30 AM

Medication Labels

The nurse is responsible to make sure that the label on the medication matches the medication in the medication order. If there is a mismatch, the nurse must not administer the medication. The pharmacy is contacted to resolve the conflict.

Some health care facilities have a policy that permits the pharmacy to substitute a generic medication for a brand name medication in consultation with the practitioner without requiring the practitioner to change the medication order.

Strength of the Medication

The medication label specifies the strength of the medication per unit of measure. This is the value that you use to calculate the dose of the medication to administer to the patient.

For example,

- A solution's strength of 30 mg/mL means each milliliter contains 30 milligrams of the medication.
- A tablet's strength of 2 mg per tablet means each tablet contains 2 milligrams of the medication.
- A capsule's strength of 10 mg per capsule means each capsule contains 10 milligrams of the medication.

Don't assume that the container holds one dose. Although many health care facilities use unit-dose packages, you must realize that not all medications come in unit-dose package.

Don't assume that the unit of strength in the medication order is the same as the unit of strength on the medication label. For example, the practitioner may specify micrograms (mcg) in the medication order and the medication label shows a strength in milligrams (mg). You'll learn how to convert these units in the next chapter.

Expiration Date

Every medication container specifies an expiration date. Always read the expiration before preparing the medication. Although the pharmacy takes every precaution to purge expired medication, outdated medication can find its way to the nursing unit.

All expired medication should be disposed of immediately according to the health care facility's policies.

NURSING ALERT

When opening a new multidose container, such as a vial of insulin, make sure you write the expiration date on the container.

CASE STUDY

CASE 1

You are the primary nurse for a 53-year-old male patient who is a new admission to the unit. The patient is admitted at 8 PM and is scheduled to have minor procedure in surgery at 7 AM. The patient is expected to be discharged by 5 PM assuming that the patient fully recovers from the procedure. You take the patient's vital signs. His blood pressure is 170/110 mm Hg. You notify the practitioner by telephone about the patient's blood pressure. What would your best response be to the following questions?

QUESTION 1. What time is written on the patient's chart to reflect when the patient admitted to your unit?

QUESTION 2. What time would you enter onto a preprocedure checklist for the minor surgical procedure?

QUESTION 3. The practitioner tells you over the phone to administer clonidine 0.1 mg. What should you do?

QUESTION 4. After you hang up the phone, your colleague reads the telephone order and asks if the practitioner ordered clonidine or klonopin. You are unsure. What should you do?

ANSWERS

1. 2000, which is military time for 8 PM.

2. 0700, which is 7 AM in military time.

3. Ask the practitioner for start and stop times and the route. Write the complete order on the health care facility's practitioner's order form and read the complete order back to the practitioner. You should sign the practitioner's order form, forward the practitioner's order form to the pharmacy, and place the practitioner's order form in the patient's chart. Make sure you flag the chart indicating that the practitioner needs to sign the practitioner's order form. The practitioner's order must be transcribed onto the patient's MAR either by pharmacist (eMAR) or by you (paper MAR). The transcription must be cosigned before the medication is administered to the patient.

4. Call the practitioner immediately to confirm the order. There are many medications that have similar sounding names. Furthermore, the telephone connection might be poor making it difficult to understand the practitioner. Never administer a medication if you are unsure of the name of the medication.

FINAL CHECK-UP

1. A nurse who is new to the unit is given a verbal STAT order for medication right before the practitioner left the unit. The nurse is unsure of the name of the medication. What is the best action to take?
   A. Ask one of the regular nurses what drug the practitioner normally orders for the patient.
   B. Call the practitioner.
   C. Review the patient's chart to see if the drug might have been previously ordered.
   D. Ask the nurse manager what drug the practitioner normally orders for the patient.

2. **The practitioner wrote and signed and dated the following order. What would you do?**

   Mark Jones Patient ID 123345, Room 1220-1, Procardia XL 30 mg p.o.

   A Calculate the dose and administer the medication.

   B. Administer the medication.

   C. Call the practitioner.

   D. None of the above.

3. **The practitioner wrote and signed and dated the following order. What would you do?**

   Mark Jones Patient ID 123345, Room 1220-1, Capoten 12.5 mg p.o. b.i.d.

   A. Calculate the dose and administer the medication.

   B. Administer the medication.

   C. Call the practitioner.

   D. None of the above.

4. **All medication orders are transcribed to the MAR by the practitioner.**

   A. True

   B. False

5. **A PRN medication order should**

   A. Specify the date and time when the medication is to be given

   B. Have the nurse manager cosigns the medication order

   C. Provide instructions to the nurse for when to give the medication

   D. Be written in front of the patient

6. **Documenting in the MAR that the medication was administered according to the medication order is done**

   A. At the beginning of the shift

   B. Immediately after the medication is administered

   C. At the end of the shift

   D. When the nurse has a free moment

7. **An example of taking off orders is the process of**

   A. Transcribing a medication order to the MAR

   B. Comparing the medication to the MAR

   C. Comparing the medication to the medication order

   D. Receiving an update about a patient at the beginning of the shift

8. A medication order is written as Q6H requiring the patient to receive the medication every 6 hours. Who determines the exact hour to give the medication?

    A. The health care facility's policy
    B. The patient
    C. The nurse manager
    D. The practitioner

9. What is the best action to take when a medication order is illegible?

    A. Call the practitioner.
    B. Ask another nurse to help read the medication order.
    C. Look up the medication in the drug book.
    D. Look up the medication in the chart.

10. How is 10 AM written in military time?

    A. 1000
    B. 010:00
    C. 10
    D. 010

CORRECT ANSWERS AND RATIONALES

1. A. Call the practitioner. Always clarify any doubt with the practitioner who wrote the order.
2. C. Call the practitioner. The order is missing the time to administer the medication.
3. A. Calculate the dose and administer the medication since the order is complete.
4. B. False. The nurse or the pharmacists transcribes medication orders to the MAR.
5. C. Provide instructions to the nurse for when to give the medication.
6. B. Immediately after the medication is administered
7. A. Transcribing a medication order to the MAR
8. A. The health care facility's policy
9. A. Call the practitioner
10. A. 1000

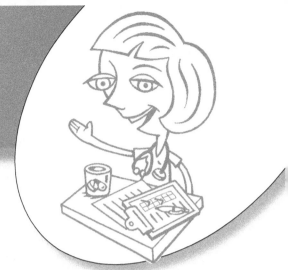

chapter 2

The Formula Method

LEARNING OBJECTIVES

1. Parts of the Formula
2. Calculating a Dose Using the Formula Method
3. Reading the Medication Order
4. Reading the Medication Label
5. Inserting Values Into the Formula
6. Calculating the Formula
7. Converting Metric Units

Based on the medical diagnosis, the practitioner prescribes a dose of the medication that will improve the patient's condition. Sometimes this is the same dose that appears on the medication label, which means that the patient receives the complete content of the container.

However, the medication might be a different dose and thus requires the nurse to calculate the amount of medication to administer to the patient.

Two methods are used to calculate the dose: the formula method and the proportion method. Both methods arrive at the same dose. Whatever method you choose, it is best to stick with it for all dose calculations to avoid errors.

In this chapter, you'll learn the formula method of calculating the dose. The proportion method is explained in the next chapter.

1. Parts of the Formula

The **formula method** has been adopted by many nurses because the formula is straightforward and easy to understand and use. If you can divide and multiply, then you won't have any trouble using the formula method.

There are following three parts to the formula:

- **Dose ordered:** The dose ordered is the dose specified in the medication order.

- **Dose on hand:** The dose on hand is the dose specified on the medication label (Figure 2–1).

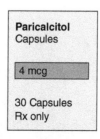

Paricalcitol
Capsules

4 mcg

30 Capsules
Rx only

FIGURE 2–1 • Here is a typical medication label that contains the quantity of medication per dose.

- **Quantity:** The quantity is the unit of measure on the medication label that contains the dose (Figure 2–1).

Writing the Formula

The secret to using the formula to calculate the dose is to properly set up the equation. The equation is written as:

$$\frac{\text{Ordered}}{\text{On hand}} \times \text{quantity} = \text{dose}$$

Some nurses use a shorter way to write this formula:

$$\frac{O}{H} \times Q = D$$

2. Calculating a Dose Using the Formula Method

There are a few steps to follow to calculate the dose using the formula method. However, avoid the trap. Be careful when performing these steps. Because these steps are simple, there is a tendency to rush through the calculations, which results in errors. Remember that an error means that you'll be giving your patient the wrong dose.

The steps are as follows:

1. Read the medication order and identify the information you need for the formula.
2. Read the medication label and identify the information you need for the formula.
3. Insert the values from the medication order and medication label into the formula.
4. Calculate.
5. Repeat steps 1 through 4 to check your answer.

3. Reading the Medication Order

The practitioner wrote the following order for Dilantin for your patient. Your job is to calculate the number of milliliters of Dilantin to give to your patient.

Dilantin 100 mg P.O. t.i.d.

What information in this order do you need to calculate the dose for your patient? Let's take apart this order.

- The name of the medication is Dilantin.
- The dose ordered is 100 mg.
- The medication is P.O. which means it is given by mouth.
- The medication is given t.i.d., which means it is given three times a day.

Only the dose ordered is needed for the calculation. Although the name of the medication must match the medication label, the name isn't used in the calculation. Likewise, you don't need to know the route and frequency of administration of the medication to calculate the dose.

4. Reading the Medication Label

The pharmacy delivered Dilantin to the unit. The following is a portion of the information contained on the label.

Dilantin suspension 125 mg/5 mL

What information on this order do you need to calculate the dose for your patient? Let's take apart this label.

- The name of the medication is Dilantin.
- The dose is 125 mg in 5 mL.

The information needed for the formula is the dose on hand, which is 125 mg, and the quantity, which is 5 mL. The name of the medication isn't required by the formula.

> **NURSING ALERT**
>
> Besides the dose, the medication label also contains the total quantity of medication in the container. Don't confuse the dose volume with the quantity in the container. In a single-dose container called a unit dose, the quantity of the medication in the container is the same as in the dose. In a multiple-dose container, the quantity is larger than the dose.

5. Inserting Values Into the Formula

Let's insert values from the medication order and the medication label into the dose calculation formula. When doing so, it is very important that you include both the value and the unit of measurement (i.e., mg, mL).

As you'll learn later in this chapter, the unit of measurement specified in the medication order may differ from the unit of measurement on the medication label. You cannot calculate unlike unit of measurements; therefore, you'll need to convert to the same unit of measurement. You'll see how this is done later in this chapter.

For now, remember to specify the unit of measurement in the formula. This will alert you if you need to convert units. In this example, the same units of measurements are used so there is no conversion.

$$\frac{100 \text{ mg}}{125 \text{ mg}} \times 5 \text{ mL} = D$$

6. Calculating the Formula

There are two mathematical operations that must be performed to calculate the dose. These are division and multiplication.

1. First divide the dose on hand into the dose ordered.

$$\frac{100 \text{ mg}}{125 \text{ mg}} = 0.8$$

2. Next, multiply by 5 mL to calculate the dose to administer to the patient.

$$0.8 \times 5 \text{ mL} = 4 \text{ mL}$$

You will administer 4 mL of Dilantin to the patient.

Rounding Tips

In the real world and on dose calculation examinations, calculated values are not always in round numbers. You will have decimal places in your calculation. Here's how you need to manage decimal places.

- Round only the final value that you calculate and leave the intermediate values unrounded. If you don't, then your answer might be incorrect although you had the values in the proper position in the formula and your math was correct.
- Round two decimal places only.
- Round only the third decimal place.

TABLE 2–1 Prefixes Used for Medication	
Prefix	**Numeric value**
Kilo	One thousand times (1000)
Centi	One hundredths of (0.01)
Milli	One thousandths of (0.001)
Micro	One millionth of (0.000001)

- Round up when the third decimal place is five or greater.
- Round down when the third decimal place is less than five.

A Close Look at the Metric System

Medication is specified using the **metric system**, which is also referred to as the **International System of Units (SI)**. There are three basic units of measurement in the metric system. These are as follows:

- **Gram:** A gram is used to measure weight.
- **Liter:** A liter is used to measure a volume.
- **Meter:** A meter is used to measure length.

Weight and volume are used in dose calculations. Length is not used to calculate a dose; however, it is used to measure a patient's height.

A **prefix** is used to identify the numeric value of the unit, that is, the number of grams, liters, and meters. Table 2–1 shows the prefixes that are commonly used in medication.

For example, a milliliter is one thousandths of a liter and a milligram is one thousandths of a gram. Table 2–2 contains abbreviations for metric units commonly used in dose calculations.

TABLE 2–2 Abbreviations of Units	
Abbreviation	**Unit**
g	gram
mg	milligram
mcg	microgram
L	liter
mL	milliliter
kg	Kilogram

7. Converting Metric Units

There will be times when the unit in the medication order will be different from the unit used on the medication label. For example, the practitioner might specify micrograms (mcg) and the label reads milligrams (mg).

This doesn't mean that the practitioner made an error or that there is a misprint on the medication label. It simply means that you must convert values to the same unit of measure before calculating the dose.

The conversion process is straightforward because you convert using a factor of 1000 and by moving the decimal point either three places to the left or right.

Let's see how this works. Say that the order is for 50 mg and the medication on hand is in micrograms. You must convert the 50 mg into micrograms before calculating the dose.

1. The first step is to determine if you are converting from a larger to a smaller amount or from a smaller to a larger amount. In this example, 50 mg is being converted to micrograms. Therefore, a larger amount (milligrams) is being converted to a smaller amount.

2. The next step is to set up the conversion equation.

   50 mg = ? mcg

3. Multiply by 1000 when converting a large value to a small value. Divide by 1000 when converting a small value to a large value. In this example, you multiply 50 mg by 1000 to convert to micrograms.

   50 mg = 50,000 mcg

A Close Look at the Apothecaries System

The **apothecaries system** is an older system for measuring weight and volume and has been widely replaced by the metric system; although some practitioners might prescribe medications using the apothecaries units. Values measured in the apothecaries system are approximations and not exact as in the metric system.

Weights are measured using grain.

- **Grain:** A grain is abbreviated as gr.

  Volume is measured in three units.

- **Minim:** A minim is abbreviated as m. Health care facilities discourage using minims.

- **Dram:** A dram is a unit used to measure dry medication. It is abbreviated as dr. Although you'll find drams on medication cup, the use of this measure has been discouraged by health care facilities.

- **Ounce:** An ounce is abbreviated as oz and is also used in the **household system** of measurement.

NURSING ALERT

Focus on learning to convert a grain to a gram and a milligram to a grain. Although you might not have to convert these units in the health care facility, you may have to convert them on a test. Also to remember is that the unit of measurement precedes the value when using grain. Here are the conversion factors to memorize.

gr 15 = 1 g
60 mg = gr 1

A Close Look at the Household System

The household system is a system of measurement used primarily for cooking and is used by patients to measure medication at home because home utensils are gauged for the household system. You'll need to convert the medication order dose from metric to household system.

The household system measures volume using the units shown in Table 2–3.

Two medications that you'll frequently need to convert to the household systems are Maalox and GoLytely. Maalox is used as an antacid and a laxative depending on the dose prescribed by the practitioner. GoLytely is a bowel

TABLE 2–3 Abbreviations of Units	
Abbreviation	**Unit**
oz	ounce
tbs or T	tablespoon
tsp or t	teaspoon
cup	cup
pt	pint
qt	quart
gal	Gallon

preparation that is prescribed prior to a colonoscopy. Both are usually taken by the patient at home.

Let's say that the practitioner wrote a medication order for Maalox 30 mL. The patient probably doesn't have a metric utensil at home to measure this amount of Maalox. Therefore, the dose must be converted to a unit of the household system.

There are following three choices:

- Two tablespoons
- Six teaspoons
- One cup

The dose for GoLytely is typically 1.2 L. The patient has a cup (8 oz) at home. You must calculate the number of cups of GoLytely that the patient must take. Looking at Table 2–4, you'll notice that there isn't a simple factor to use to convert liters to a cup. Therefore, you'll need to perform intermediate conversions.

TABLE 2–4 Conversion Factors From Metric to the Household System
1 oz = 30 mL
1 tbs = 15 mL
1 tsp = 5 mL
1 cup = 240 mL = 8 oz
1 pt = 500 mL = 32 oz
1 qt = 1000 mL = 32 oz
1 gal = 4 qt

Here's how to perform this conversion.

1. Convert 1.2 L into milliliters. You're going from large to small so move the decimal point three positions to the right.

   1.2 L = 1200 mL

2. Convert 1200 mL to cups. Table 2–4 states that 240 mL equals 1 cup. Therefore, dividing 1200 mL by 240 mL will result in the number of cups GoLytely the patient needs to take.

$$\frac{1200 \text{ mL}}{240 \text{ mL}} = 5 \text{ cups}$$

CASE STUDY

CASE 1

Calculate the correct dose for the following orders.

QUESTION 1. Medication order: Capoten 6.25 mg P.O. q8h
Medication label: Capoten 12.5 mg per tablet
How many tablets to administer to the patient?

QUESTION 2. Medication order: Morphine sulfate 2 mg I.M. STAT
Medication label: Morphine sulfate 10 mg/mL
How many milliliters to administer to the patient?

QUESTION 3. Medication order: Xanax 0.25 mg P.O. daily
Medication label: Xanax 0.5 mg per tablet
How many tablets to administer to the patient?

QUESTION 4. Medication order: Charcotabs 520 mg P.O. STAT
Medication label: Charcotabs 260 mg per tablet
How many tablets to administer to the patient?

QUESTION 5. Medication order: Demerol 75 mg I.M. PRN
Medication label: Demerol 50 mg/mL
How many milliliters to administer to the patient?

QUESTION 6. Medication order: Allopurinol 300 mg P.O. daily
Medication label: Allopurinol 100 mg per tablet
How many tablets to administer to the patient?

QUESTION 7. Medication order: Garamycin 60 mg I.M. STAT
Medication label: Garamycin 80 mg/mL
How many milliliters to administer to the patient?

QUESTION 8. Medication order: Corophyllin 500 mg q6h
Medication label: Corophyllin 250 mg/1 rectal suppository
How many tablets to administer to the patient?

QUESTION 9. Medication order: Colace 50 mg P.O. daily
Medication label: Colace 100 mg/capsule
How many capsules to administer to the patient?

QUESTION 10. Medication order: Azulfidine 1000 mg P.O. daily
Medication label: Azulfidine 500 mg per tablet
How many tablets to administer to the patient?

ANSWERS

1. $\dfrac{6.25 \text{ mg}}{12.5 \text{ mg}} \times 1 \text{ tablet} = 0.5 \text{ tablet}$

2. $\dfrac{2 \text{ mg}}{10 \text{ mg}} \times 1 \text{ mL} = 0.2 \text{ mL}$

3. $\dfrac{0.25 \text{ mg}}{0.5 \text{ mg}} \times 1 \text{ tablet} = 0.5 \text{ tablet}$

4. $\dfrac{520 \text{ mg}}{260 \text{ mg}} \times 1 \text{ tablet} = 2 \text{ tablets}$

5. $\dfrac{75 \text{ mg}}{50 \text{ mg}} \times 1 \text{ mL} = 1.5 \text{ mL}$

6. $\dfrac{300 \text{ mg}}{100 \text{ mg}} \times 1 \text{ tablet} = 3 \text{ tablets}$

7. $\dfrac{60 \text{ mg}}{80 \text{ mg}} \times 1 \text{ mL} = 0.75 \text{ mL}$

8. $\dfrac{500 \text{ mg}}{250 \text{ mg}} \times 1 \text{ rectal suppository} = 2 \text{ rectal suppositories}$

9. $\dfrac{50 \text{ mg}}{100 \text{ mg}} \times 1 \text{ capsule} = 0.5 \text{ capsule}$

10. $\dfrac{1000 \text{ mg}}{500 \text{ mg}} \times 1 \text{ tablet} = 2 \text{ tablets}$

CASE STUDY

CASE 2

Calculate the correct dose for the following orders. Make sure to convert the necessary units.

QUESTION 1. Medication order: Vitamin B12 1 mg P.O. daily
Medication label: Vitamin B12 500 mcg per tablet
How many tablets to administer to the patient?

QUESTION 2. Medication order: Erythromycin 100 mg I.V.
Medication label: Erythromycin 1 g/30 mL
How many milliliters to administer to the patient?

QUESTION 3. Medication order: Methozamine HCl 0.015 g I.M. daily
Medication label: Methozamine HCl 10 mg/mL
How many milliliters to administer to the patient?

QUESTION 4. Medication order: Quinidine Sulfate 400 mg P.O. daily
Medication Label: Quinidine Sulfate 0.2 g per tablet
How many tablets to administer to the patient?

QUESTION 5. Medication order: Lopid 0.6 g P.O. daily
Medication label: Lopid 600 mg per tablet
How many tablets to administer to the patient?

QUESTION 6. Medication order: Amphojet 5 mL P.O. daily
The patient has a teaspoon available at home.
How many teaspoons should the patient take of Amphojet?

QUESTION 7. Medication order: Maalox 1 oz P.O. daily
The patient has a tablespoon available at home.
How many tablespoons should the patient take of Maalox?

QUESTION 8. Medication order: Water 1 gal P.O. daily
The patient has an 8 oz cup available at home.
How many cups should the patient take of water?

QUESTION 9. Medication order: Milk of Magnesia 30 mL P.O. daily
The patient has a tablespoon available at home.
How many tablespoons should the patient take of Milk of Magnesia?

QUESTION 10. Medication order: Fruit juice 4000 mL P.O. daily
The patient has 1 qt container available at home.
How many quarts should the patient take of fruit juice?

ANSWERS

1. Convert milligrams (mg) to micrograms (mcg) because the medication on hand is in micrograms.

$$1\,mg \times 1000 = 1000\,mcg$$

   Calculate the dose

$$\frac{1000\,mg}{500\,mcg} \times 1\,tablet = 2\,tablets$$

2. Convert milligrams (mg) to grams (g) because the medication on hand is in grams.

$$\frac{100\,mg}{1000} = 0.1\,g$$

   Calculate the dose

$$\frac{0.1\,g}{1\,g} \times 30\,mL = 3\,mL$$

3. Convert grams (g) to milligrams (mg) because the medication is in milligrams.

$$0.015\,g \times 1000 = 15\,mg$$

   Calculate the dose

$$\frac{15\,mg}{10\,mg} \times 1\,mL = 1.5\,mL$$

4. Convert milligrams (mg) to grams (g) because the medication on hand is in grams.

$$\frac{400\,mg}{1000} = 0.4\,g$$

   Calculate the dose

$$\frac{0.4\,g}{0.2\,g} \times 1\,tablet = 2\,tablets$$

5. Convert grams (g) to milligrams (mg) because the medication is in milligrams

$$0.6\,g \times 1000 = 600\,mg$$

   Calculate the dose

$$\frac{600\,mg}{600\,mg} \times 1\,tablet = 1\,tablet$$

6. $5\,mL = 1$ teaspoon

7. 1 oz = 30 mL

   1 tablespoon = 15 mL

$$\frac{30 \text{ mL}}{15 \text{ mL}} = 2 \text{ tablespoons}$$

8. 1 gal = 4 qt

   1 qt = 32 oz

   4 qt × 32 oz = 128 oz = 1 gal

$$\frac{128 \text{ oz}}{8 \text{ oz}} = 16 \text{ cups}$$

9. 1 tablespoon = 15 mL

$$\frac{30 \text{ mL}}{15 \text{ mL}} = 2 \text{ tablespoons}$$

10. 1 qt = 1000 mL

$$\frac{4000 \text{ mL}}{1000 \text{ mL}} = 4 \text{ qt}$$

FINAL CHECK-UP

1. The medication order is for Lanoxin 0.50 mg and the pharmacy delivered Lanoxin 0.25 mg per tablet. What dose would you administer to the patient?

   A. 2 tablets

   B. A half of a tablet

   C. 1 tablet

   D. 2.5 tablets

2. The medication order is for Motrin 0.6 g and the pharmacy delivered Motrin 400 mg per tablet. What dose would you administer to the patient?

   A. 1 tablet

   B. 1.25 tablets

   C. 1.5 tablets

   D. 0.5 tablets

3. The medication order is for Decadron 3 mg and the pharmacy delivered Decadron 0.75 mg per tablet. What dose would you administer to the patient?

   A. 2.5 tablets

   B. 2 tablets

   C. 4 tablets

   D. 4.5 tablets

4. The medication order is for Milk of Magnesia 5 mL. You should tell the patient to use 1 teaspoon of Milk of Magnesia.

   A. True
   B. False

5. The medication order is for Norpace 0.30 g and the pharmacy delivered Norpace 150 mg per tablet. What dose would you administer to the patient?

   A. 2.5 tablets
   B. 2 tablets
   C. 3 tablets
   D. 3.5 tablets

6. The medication order is for Vistaril 25 mg and the pharmacy delivered Vistaril 50 mg/mL. What dose would you administer to the patient?

   A. 2.5 mL
   B. 2 mL
   C. 1 mL
   D. 0.5 mL

7. The medication order is for Ampicillin 1 g and the pharmacy delivered Ampicillin 500 mg per capsule. What dose would you administer to the patient?

   A. 2.5 capsules
   B. 2 capsules
   C. 3 capsules
   D. 3.5 capsules

8. The medication order is for Dilantin 50 mg and the pharmacy delivered Dilantin 125 mg/5 mL. What dose would you administer to the patient?

   A. 2 mL
   B. 2.5 mL
   C. 3 mL
   D. 4.5 mL

9. The medication order is for Synthroid 0.05 mg and the pharmacy delivered Synthroid 25 mcg per tablet. What dose would you administer to the patient?

   A. 2 tablets
   B. 2.5 tablets
   C. 3 tablets
   D. 3.5 tablets

10. The medication order is for Demerol 50 mg and the pharmacy delivered Demerol 75 mg per mL. What dose would you administer to the patient?

A. 0.60 mL

B. 0.66 mL

C. 0.67 mL

D. 0.70 mL

CORRECT ANSWERS AND RATIONALES

1. A. 2 tablets
2. C. 1.5 tablets
3. C. 4 tablets
4. A. True
5. B. 2 tablets
6. D. 0.5 mL
7. B. 2 capsules
8. A. 2 mL
9. A. 2 tablets
10. C. 0.67 mL

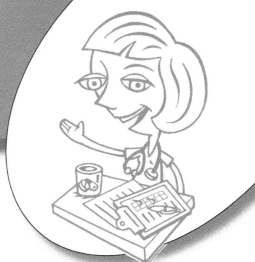

chapter 3

The Ratio-Proportion Method

LEARNING OBJECTIVES

1. Understanding the Ratio
2. Proportion
3. Ratio

KEY TERMS

Calculating Using the Ratio-
  Proportional Expression
Points to Remember When Using the
  Ratio-Proportional Expression

The Ratio-Proportion Expression

Ratio-proportion is another method used for calculating the dose to administer to patient. It is similar to the formula method that you learned in Chapter 2. Both methods arrive at the same dose. Only the calculation is different.

The goal of the ratio-proportion method is to solve for X using a simple algebraic expression. X is the dose. Other elements of the expression are given in the medication order and on the medication label.

You'll learn how to use the ratio-proportion method in this chapter and be in the position to choose the ratio-proportion method or the formula method to calculate the dose of medication for your patients.

1. Understanding the Ratio

Before diving into math, step back a moment and take another look at the dose on a medication label.

$$25 \text{ mg/mL}$$

This is saying that every milliliter of fluid contains 25 mg of medication. In other words if you draw up 1 mL from the container into a syringe, the syringe will have 25 mg of medication.

Suppose you drew up 2 mL into the syringe. How many milligrams of medication are in the syringe? You probably answered this in your head because intuitively you realize if the quantity (mL) doubled so must the amount of medication (mg). There are 50 mg of medication in the syringe.

Intuitively you used ratio-proportion to calculate the dose.

2. Proportion

Proportion means there is a linear relationship between two values. This simply means that an increase in one value causes the other value to increase at the same rate. This relationship between the dose and quantity is printed on the medication label.

The pharmaceutical that made the medication determined the proportion through research and clinical trials that occur before the Food and Drug Administration approved the medication for clinical use.

3. Ratio

A **ratio** is a way to write the proportional relationship of two values. There are two ways that you'll see a ratio written. The first is the way the ratio appears on the medication label such as

25 mg/mL

The other way is to write the ratio in an expression using the colon instead of the forward slash such as

25 mg/mL

Both of these are saying the same thing, that is, there are 25 mg in each milliliter of fluid in the container.

The Ratio-Proportion Expression

The ratio-proportion expression is divided into two components: known and unknown. The known component is the ratio on the medication label. The unknown component is the medication order.

As you'll recall from the last chapter, the medication order specifies a dose but not the quantity. You must calculate the quantity.

Let's say that physician ordered 50 mg of a medication. The medication label reads 100 mg/mL. Here's how to represent this in the ratio-proportion expression.

100 mg: 1 mL = 50 mg: X mL

The known (medication label), the left of the equal sign, is a ratio. The unknown (medication order), to the right of the equal sign, is also a ratio except an X is used to represent the quantity. The objective is to solve X.

The proportional relationship between the dose and the quantity of the medication label is the key to calculating the dose. You apply this proportion to the unknown side of the ratio-proportion expression to determine the dose to administer to the patient.

Calculating Using the Ratio-Proportional Expression

The initial step in calculating the ratio-proportional expression is to transform the ratio-proportional expression into two fractions by replacing the colon with a division sign as shown here:

$$\frac{100 \text{ mg}}{1 \text{ mL}} = \frac{50 \text{ mg}}{X \text{ mL}}$$

The next step is to cross multiply. When cross multiplying, apply the rules of algebra and move values from the left side of the expression to the right side so that X is on the left side of the expression. When a value is moved, its operation is reversed.

Move 100 mg to the right side and X mL to the left side as shown here:

$$\frac{X \text{ mL}}{1 \text{ mL}} = \frac{50 \text{ mg}}{100 \text{ mg}}$$

Next, move 1 mL to the right side of the expression. The operation on the left side of the expression is division; therefore, the operation is reversed to multiplication when the 1 mL quantity is moved to the right side of the expression as shown here:

$$X \text{ mL} = \frac{50 \text{ mg}}{100 \text{ mg}} \times 1 \text{ mL}$$

The last step is to calculate the expression.

$$X \text{ mL} = 0.5 \times 1 \text{ mL}$$
$$X \text{ mL} = 0.5 \text{ mL}$$

Points to Remember When Using the Ratio-Proportional Expression

- The known (medication label) ratio is on the left of the equal sign and the unknown (medication order) is on the right.
- Set up each ratio the same way—dose:quantity
- Always label each value in each ratio.
- Make sure like units of measurements are used. If the unit of measurement in the medication order is different from the unit of measurement on the medication label, then convert the medication order to the medication label unit of measurement.
- Only round the value of X. Don't round intermediate values.
- X must be the lone value to the left of the equal sign.

CASE STUDY

CASE 1

Calculate the correct dose for the following orders from Chapter 2 using the ratio-proportion method.

QUESTION 1. Medication order: Capoten 6.25 mg P.O. q8h
Medication label: Capoten 12.5 mg per tablet
How many tablets to administer to the patient?

QUESTION 2. Medication order: Morphine sulfate 2 mg I.M. STAT
Medication label: Morphine sulfate 10 mg/mL
How many milliliters to administer to the patient?

QUESTION 3. Medication order: Xanax 0.25 mg P.O. daily
Medication label: Xanax 0.5 mg per tablet
How many tablets to administer to the patient?

QUESTION 4. Medication order: Charcotabs 520 mg P.O. STAT
Medication label: Charcotabs 260 mg per tablet
How many tablets to administer to the patient?

QUESTION 5. Medication order: Demerol 75 mg I.M. PRN
Medication label: Demerol 50 mg/mL
How many milliliters to administer to the patient?

QUESTION 6. Medication order: Allopurinol 300 mg P.O. daily
Medication label: Allopurinol 100 mg per tablet
How many tablets to administer to the patient?

QUESTION 7. Medication order: Garamycin 60 mg I.M. STAT
Medication label: Garamycin 80 mg/mL
How many milliliters to administer to the patient?

QUESTION 8. Medication order: Corophyllin 500 mg q6h
Medication label: Corophyllin 250 mg/1 rectal suppository
How many tablets to administer to the patient?

QUESTION 9. Medication order: Colace 50 mg P.O. daily
Medication label: Colace 100 mg/capsule
How many capsules to administer to the patient?

QUESTION 10. Medication order: Azulfidine 1000 mg P.O. daily
Medication label: Azulfidine 500 mg per tablet
How many tablets to administer to the patient?

ANSWERS

1. $\dfrac{12.5\,\text{mg}}{1\,\text{tablet}} = \dfrac{6.25\,\text{mg}}{X\,\text{tablet}}$

$\dfrac{X\,\text{tablet}}{1\,\text{tablet}} = \dfrac{6.25\,\text{mg}}{12.5\,\text{mg}}$

$X\,\text{tablet} = \dfrac{6.25\,\text{mg}}{12.5\,\text{mg}} \times 1\,\text{tablet}$

$X\,\text{tablet} = 0.5 \times 1\,\text{tablet}$

$X\,\text{tablet} = 0.5\,\text{tablet}$

2. $\dfrac{10\,\text{mg}}{1\,\text{mL}} = \dfrac{2\,\text{mg}}{X\,\text{mL}}$

$\dfrac{X\,\text{mL}}{1\,\text{mL}} = \dfrac{2\,\text{mg}}{10\,\text{mg}}$

$X\,\text{mL} = \dfrac{2\,\text{mg}}{10\,\text{mg}} \times 1\,\text{mL}$

$X\,\text{mL} = 0.2 \times 1\,\text{mL}$

$X\,\text{mL} = 0.2\,\text{mL}$

3. $\dfrac{0.5\,\text{mg}}{1\,\text{tablet}} = \dfrac{0.25\,\text{mg}}{X\,\text{tablet}}$

$\dfrac{X\,\text{tablet}}{1\,\text{tablet}} = \dfrac{0.25\,\text{mg}}{0.5\,\text{mg}}$

$X\,\text{tablet} = \dfrac{0.25\,\text{mg}}{0.5\,\text{mg}} \times 1\,\text{tablet}$

$X\,\text{tablet} = 0.5 \times 1\,\text{tablet}$

$X\,\text{tablet} = 0.5\,\text{tablet}$

4. $\dfrac{260\,\text{mg}}{1\,\text{tablet}} = \dfrac{520\,\text{mg}}{X\,\text{tablet}}$

$\dfrac{X\,\text{tablet}}{1\,\text{tablet}} = \dfrac{520\,\text{mg}}{260\,\text{mg}}$

$X\,\text{tablet} = \dfrac{520\,\text{mg}}{260\,\text{mg}} \times 1\,\text{tablet}$

$X\,\text{tablet} = 2 \times 1\,\text{tablet}$

$X\,\text{tablet} = 2\,\text{tablets}$

5. $\dfrac{50\,mg}{1\,mL}=\dfrac{75\,mg}{X\,mL}$

$\dfrac{X\,mL}{1\,mL}=\dfrac{75\,mg}{50\,mg}$

$X\,mL=\dfrac{75\,mg}{50\,mg}\times1\,mL$

$X\,mL=1.5\times1\,mL$

$X\,mL=1.5\ mL$

6. $\dfrac{100\,mg}{1\,tablet}=\dfrac{300\,mg}{X\,tablet}$

$\dfrac{X\,tablet}{1\,tablet}=\dfrac{300\,mg}{100\,mg}$

$X\,tablet=\dfrac{300\,mg}{100\,mg}\times1\,tablet$

$X\,tablet=3\times1\,tablet$

$X\,tablet=3\ tablets$

7. $\dfrac{80\,mg}{1\,mL}=\dfrac{60\,mg}{X\,mL}$

$\dfrac{X\,mL}{1\,mL}=\dfrac{60\,mg}{80\,mg}$

$X\,mL=\dfrac{60\,mg}{80\,mg}\times1\,mL$

$X\,mL=0.75\times1\,mL$

$X\,mL=0.75\ mL$

8. $\dfrac{250\,mg}{1\,rectal\ suppository}=\dfrac{500\,mg}{X\,rectal\ suppository}$

$\dfrac{X\,rectal\ suppository}{1\,rectal\ suppository}=\dfrac{500\,mg}{250\,mg}$

$X\,rectal\ suppository=\dfrac{500\,mg}{250\,mg}\times1\,rectal\ suppository$

$X\,rectal\ suppository=2\times1\,rectal\ suppository$

$X\,rectal\ suppository=2\ rectal\ suppositories$

$$\frac{100\,mg}{1\,capsule} = \frac{50\,mg}{X\,capsule}$$

$$\frac{X\,capsule}{1\,capsule} = \frac{50\,mg}{100\,mg}$$

$$X\,capsule = \frac{50\,mg}{100\,mg} \times 1\,capsule$$

$$X\,capsule = 0.5 \times 1\,capsule$$

$$X\,capsule = 0.5\,capsule$$

9.

10.
$$\frac{500\,mg}{1\,tablet} = \frac{1000\,mg}{X\,tablet}$$

$$\frac{X\,tablet}{1\,tablet} = \frac{1000\,mg}{500\,mg}$$

$$X\,tablet = \frac{1000\,mg}{500\,mg} \times 1\,tablet$$

$$X\,tablet = 2 \times 1\,tablet$$

$$X\,tablet = 2\,tablets$$

FINAL CHECK-UP

1. The medication order is for Guaifenesin 100 mg and the pharmacy delivered Guaifenesin 200 mg/5 mL. What dose would you administer to the patient?

   A. 2 mL

   B. 2.5 mL

   C. 1 mL

   D. 1.5 mL

2. The medication order is for Valproic 1.5 mg and the pharmacy delivered Valproic 3 mg/mL. What dose would you administer to the patient?

   A. 1 mL

   B. 1.25 mL

   C. 1.5 mL

   D. 0.5 mL

3. The medication order is for Xanax 4000 mcg and the pharmacy delivered Xanax 2 mg/tablet. What dose would you administer to the patient?

   A. 2.5 tablets

   B. 2 tablets

   C. 4 tablets

   D. 4.5 tablets

4. The medication order is for Dimelor 2.5 mg. The medication label reads Dimelor 5 mg/tablet. You should administer a half of tablet.

   A. True
   B. False

5. The medication order is for Demerol 75 mg and the pharmacy delivered Demerol 25 mg/0.5 mL. What dose would you administer to the patient?

   A. 1.5 mL
   B. 1 mL
   C. 2 mL
   D. 2.5 mL

6. The medication order is for Chloral Hydrate 50 mg and the pharmacy delivered Chloral Hydrate 25 mg/2 mL. What dose would you administer to the patient?

   A. 3 mL
   B. 3.5 mL
   C. 4 mL
   D. 4.5 mL

7. The medication order is for Norvasc 500 mg and the pharmacy delivered Norvasc 250 mg/tablet. What dose would you administer to the patient?

   A. 2.5 capsules
   B. 2 capsules
   C. 3 capsules
   D. 3.5 capsules

8. The medication order is for Keflex 250 mg and the pharmacy delivered Keflex 125 mg/capsule. What dose would you administer to the patient?

   A. 1 capsule
   B. 1.5 capsules
   C. 2 capsules
   D. 2.5 capsules

9. The medication order is for Allopurinol 105 mg and the pharmacy delivered Allopurinol 30 mg/tablet. What dose would you administer to the patient?

   A. 2 tablets
   B. 2.5 tablets
   C. 3 tablets
   D. 3.5 tablets

10. The medication order is for Azulfidine 250 mg and the pharmacy delivered Azulfidine 50 mg/tablet. What dose would you administer to the patient?

   A. 4 tablets
   B. 4.5 tablets
   C. 5 tablets
   D. 5.5 tablets

CORRECT ANSWERS AND RATIONALES

1. B. 2.5 mL
2. D. 0.5 mL
3. B. 2 tablets
4. A. True
5. A. 1.5 mL
6. C. 4 mL
7. B. 2 capsules
8. C. 2 capsules
9. D. 3.5 tablets
10. C. 5 tablets

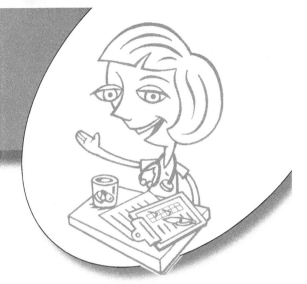

chapter *4*

Intravenous Calculations

LEARNING OBJECTIVES

1. Understanding Intravenous Therapy
2. Electronic Medication Pump
3. The Intravenous Bag
4. The Drip Factor
5. Parts of the Drip Rate Formula
6. Pump Rate

KEY TERMS

Calculating How Much Longer the
   Intravenous Will Run
Calculating the Drip Rate
Calculating the Pump Rate
Reading the Intravenous Medication
   Order

Setting the Drip Rate
The Drip Rate Formula
The Pump Rate Formula

Your patient may require intravenous (I.V.) therapy, which is a continuous flow of medication delivered into the patient's vein over a period of time. How much medication the patient receives depends on the rate of flow of the I.V.

The rate is controlled by setting the number of drops of fluid that are administered to the patient each minute. Alternatively, the rate is controlled by the number of milliliters delivered each hour to the patient by a medication pump.

The medication order specifies the medication, the volume, and the time period within which the medication is infused into the patient. You calculate the number of drops or the milliliters setting for the medication pump. You'll learn how to perform these calculations in this chapter.

1. Understanding Intravenous Therapy

The primary goal of I.V. therapy is to deliver medication to the patient quickly. The medication is immediately delivered to the bloodstream where it circulates throughout the body. There isn't any delay as with an intramuscular injection or with administering medication orally, which requires the medication to be absorbed into the bloodstream.

The medication is contained in either a plastic bag or a glass bottle. Tubing connects the bag to the lock, which is attached to the patient's vein. The tubing has a **drip chamber** and a **roller clamp**. The drip chamber is a clear cylinder used to view drops of medication from the bag. The roller clamp is used to control the number of drops of medication per minute that enters the tube from the drip chamber. After calculating the **drip rate**, you use the roller clamp to set the drip rate of the I.V.

2. Electronic Medication Pump

The health care facility may require that some or all I.V. medications be administered using an **electronic medication pump**. The pump controls the flow of medication that the patient receives.

Tubing is still used to connect the bag to the lock; however, a portion of the tubing is placed within the pump. The pump takes the place of the roller clamp in controlling the rate of medication received by the patient. The roller clamp is totally open when the pump is used.

The delivery rate on the pump is specified in milliliters/hour for a specific length of time. The medication order specifies the number of milliliters and over what period of time it is to be delivered. You must calculate the hourly rate and then enter the rate into the pump.

Reading the Intravenous Medication Order

In addition to the required elements of a medication order (see Chapter 1), there are three components unique to an I.V. Every I.V. order must have these components; otherwise the medication order is invalid and should not be administered.

Intravenous Solution

The physician must tell you the name of this medication. The order might also have the name of medications that must be added to the I.V. solution depending on the physician's course of treatment.

Volume

This is the amount of the solution that the patient is to receive usually specified in milliliters. It is important to realize that the volume specified in the order may be less than the volume specified on the I.V. bag. Therefore, you base your calculation on the volume ordered by the physician and not the volume on the I.V. bag. You will likely to see questions that show both the volume of the bag and the volume ordered. You must decide which volume to use in your calculation.

Infusion Time

This specifies the time period to give the volume of medication to the patient. The time is commonly ordered as half hour or in hours. Sometimes the time can be in minutes such as within a 15-minute period.

3. The Intravenous Bag

The I.V. bag label contains the name of the medication and the volume contained in the I.V. bag. It also contains text that provides details of the solution including the ratio of medication per 100 mL of I.V. fluid. You don't use this ratio in your flow rate calculation.

At the top of the I.V. bag is a lot number and expiration date. The lot number identifies when the solution was produced. The expiration date is similar to the expiration date on other medications that you learned about in Chapter 1. If the solution has expired, then don't use it.

Numbers along the side of the bag are used to measure the volume of solution infused into the patient. Each represents 100 mL.

The Drip Rate Formula

The drip rate formula is used to calculate the number of drops per minute of the medication that the patient is to receive. This is the number of drops that appears in the drip chamber in a minute.

Here's an example of a medication order for I.V. therapy.

1000 mL D5W I.V. in 8 hours

In order to calculate the drip rate, you need to know:

The **drip factor** of the tubing

Total volume

Number of minutes of the infusion

4. The Drip Factor

The drip factor is the number of drops that equals 1 mL. The drip factor depends on the tubing that is used for the infusion and is specified on the bag that contains the tubing. The drip factor is written as gtt/mL where **gtt** is the abbreviation for drop.

For example, the bag containing the I.V. tubing might have 10 gtt/mL on the bag. This is the drip factor for the tubing that you use to calculate the drip rate for the I.V. medication. If you don't see a drip factor on the bag, then don't use the tubing.

There are two categories of drip factors. These are **macrodrops** and **microdrops.** Macrodrop tubing typically has 10, 15, or 20 gtt/mL. Microdrop tubing always has 60 gtt/mL as the drip factor.

> **NURSING ALERT**
>
> If you see macrodrop on the bag, then use 60 gtt/mL as the drip factor. Macrodrop tubing always has the drip factor marked on the bag.

5. Parts of the Drip Rate Formula

There are several different formulas that can be used to calculate the drip rate. Here's the formula that is commonly used:

$$X \text{ gtt/min} = \frac{\text{Volume ordered} \times \text{Drip factor}}{\text{Minutes to infuse}}$$

The value for the volume ordered is found on the medication order. The drip factor is on the I.V. bag. The minutes to infuse the medication are also on the medication order, but this is usually stated as hours or half hour.

Calculating the Drip Rate

Let's calculate the drip rate for the following medication order. Assume that you are using macrodrop tubing with a 10 gtt/mL drip factor.

1000 mL D5W I.V. in 8 hours

1. Convert the **infusion time** from 8 hours to minutes because the drip rate is in minutes.

$$480 \text{ minutes} = 8 \text{ hours} \times 60 \text{ minutes}$$

2. Place values into the formula.

$$X \text{ gtt/min} = \frac{1000 \text{ mL} \times 10 \text{ gtt/mL}}{480 \text{ minutes}}$$

3. Calculate the total number of drops in the volume.

$$X \text{ gtt/min} = \frac{10,000 \text{ gtt}}{480 \text{ minutes}}$$

4. Calculate the number of drops per minute.

$$20.833 \text{ gtt/min} = \frac{10,000 \text{ gtt}}{480 \text{ minutes}}$$

5. Round to the whole number. Remember these are drops. You can't set the drip rate to a fraction of a drop. Round up if the value is 5 or greater. Round down if the value is less than 5.

$$21 \text{ gtt/min}$$

Setting the Drip Rate

Now that you calculated the drip rate, you must set this rate using the I.V. tubing roller clamp. You do this by adjusting the roller clamp so that the calculated number of drops fall through the drip chamber each minute. This is 21 drops/min in the previous example.

Setting the drip rate can be tricky because you have to keep one eye on the drip chamber and another on the clock. A method used by some nurses makes this a straightforward process. Hold your watch next to the drip chamber so both are in the same view.

NURSING ALERT

Another trick is to calculate the number of drips for less than a minute. Say that the drip rate per minute is 60 gtt. This also means there are 6 gtt per 10 seconds. You need only to see 6 drops within 10 seconds in the drip chamber to set the correct drip rate rather than counting drops for a full minute.

---

6. Pump Rate

There is a tendency of health care facilities to use an electronic medication pump rather than the drip method to control the flow of the medication to the patient. Some medications must be delivered using the electronic medication pump because the flow rate must be accurately metered.

Although there are various kinds of electronic medication pumps used by health care facilities, most require three settings. These are the total volume in the bag or bottle, the total length of time of the infusion, and the number of milliliters that are to be infused per hour.

The total volume and the total length of time of the infusion are found in the medication order. You calculate the number of milliliters that are to be infused per hour.

Based on these settings, electronic sensors in the electronic medication pump administer the prescribed dose and stop the flow automatically when the prescribed dose is given. An alarm sounds when the pump stops. This happens whenever the flow stops including if there is a kink in the tube.

The Pump Rate Formula

The pump rate formula has following two components:

Volume: This is the volume in milliliters specified in the medication order.

Time: This is the time in hours specified in the medication order. Pumps will also accept time in minutes.

Here is how to construct the pump rate formula:

$$mL/hr = \frac{volume\ mL}{time\ hr}$$

Calculating the Pump Rate

Let's say you received the following medication order:

1000 mL normal saline I.V. over 12 hours

An electronic medication pump is available, so you'll need to calculate the volume of normal saline that is to be administered to the patient every hour.

1. Enter the values from the medication order into the formula.

$$mL/hr = \frac{1000\ mL}{12\ hr}$$

2. Calculate the formula.

$$mL/hr = 83.333$$

3. The pump accepts only whole numbers. Therefore, any decimal values must be rounded. Round up if the decimal value is 5 or greater and round down if the decimal value is less than 5. This is the value that you enter into the pump.

$$mL/hr = 83$$

Calculating How Much Longer the Intravenous Will Run

You might find that your patient is receiving I.V. medication started by the previous shift and you'll need to know how much time is left before the infusion is completed. This is handy to know so you can schedule your time to care for this and other patients.

You calculate the remaining time by knowing the milliliter per hour setting for the pump and the current volume in the bag.

Here's the formula to use:

$$Time\ remaining = \frac{current\ volume\ (mL)}{pump\ setting\ (mL)}$$

Say that your patient has received 150 mL of Lactated Ringers I.V. and the I.V. bag currently has a volume of 100 mL of Lactated Ringers. The pump is set at 30 mL/hr. How much longer does the infusion have to run?

1. Insert the values into the formula.

$$\text{Time remaining} = \frac{50 \text{ mL}}{30 \text{ mL}}$$

2. Divide the current volume by the pump setting.

$$\text{Time remaining} = 1.66 \text{ hours}$$

3. Convert the decimal value to minutes.

$$\text{Minutes} = 60 \text{ minutes} \times 0.66 = 39.6 \text{ minutes} = 40 \text{ minutes}$$

4. Time remaining = 1 hour 40 minutes

NURSING ALERT

You only need to estimate the time remaining for the infusion.

CASE STUDY

CASE 1
Calculate the correct drip rate for the following orders.

QUESTION 1. Medication order: 1000 mL normal saline I.V. at 40 mL/hr
Use tubing with a 15 gtt/mL drip factor
What is the drip rate?

QUESTION 2. Medication order: 1 L normal saline I.V. over 12 hours
Use tubing with a 10 gtt/mL drip factor
What is the drip rate?

QUESTION 3. Medication order: Cefadyl 5 g diluted in 100 mL of normal saline I.V. over a half hour
Use tubing with a 10 gtt/mL drip factor
What is the drip rate?

QUESTION 4. Medication order: Gentamycin 2 g diluted in 100 mL of normal saline I.V. over 1 hour
Use tubing with a 15 gtt/mL drip factor
What is the drip rate?

QUESTION 5. Medication order: 1000 mL normal saline I.V. over 15 hours
Use tubing with a 15 gtt/mL drip factor
What is the drip rate?

QUESTION 6. Medication order: 1000 mL of 0.9% of sodium chloride I.V. over 60 mL/hr
Use tubing with a 10 gtt/mL drip factor
What is the drip rate?

QUESTION 7. Medication order: 500 mL Ringers Lactate I.V. over 6 hours
Use tubing with a 10 gtt/mL drip factor
What is the drip rate?

QUESTION 8. Medication order: 25 mL normal saline I.V. over 30 minutes
Use tubing with a 15 gtt/mL drip factor
What is the drip rate?

QUESTION 9. Medication order: 1000 mL Ringers Lactate I.V. over 5 hours
Use microdrip tubing
What is the drip rate?

QUESTION 10. Medication order: 2000 mL of 0.9% of sodium chloride I.V. over 24 hours
Use tubing with a 10 gtt/mL drip factor
What is the drip rate?

ANSWERS

1. 60 minutes = 1 hour

$$X \text{ gtt/min} = \frac{40 \text{ mL} \times 15 \text{ gtt/mL}}{60 \text{ minutes}}$$

$$X \text{ gtt/min} = \frac{600 \text{ gtt}}{60 \text{ minutes}}$$

$$= 10 \text{ gtt/min}$$

2.   1000 mL = 1 L × 1000

720 minutes = 12 hours × 60 minutes

$$X \text{ gtt/min} = \frac{1000 \text{ mL} \times 10 \text{ gtt/mL}}{720 \text{ minutes}}$$

$$X \text{ gtt/min} = \frac{10,000 \text{ gtt}}{720 \text{ minutes}}$$

$$= 13.888 \text{ gtt/min}$$

$$= 14 \text{ gtt/min}$$

3. $X \text{ gtt/min} = \dfrac{100 \text{ mL} \times 10 \text{ gtt/mL}}{30 \text{ minutes}}$

   $X \text{ gtt/min} = \dfrac{1000 \text{ gtt}}{30 \text{ minutes}}$

   $= 33.333 \text{ gtt/min}$

   $= 33 \text{ gtt/min}$

4. $60 \text{ minutes} = 1 \text{ hour}$

   $X \text{ gtt/min} = \dfrac{100 \text{ mL} \times 15 \text{ gtt/mL}}{60 \text{ minutes}}$

   $X \text{ gtt/min} = \dfrac{1500 \text{ gtt}}{60 \text{ minutes}}$

   $= 25 \text{ gtt/min}$

5. $900 \text{ minutes} = 15 \text{ hours} \times 60 \text{ minutes}$

   $X \text{ gtt/min} = \dfrac{1000 \text{ mL} \times 15 \text{ gtt/mL}}{900 \text{ minutes}}$

   $X \text{ gtt/min} = \dfrac{15{,}000 \text{ gtt}}{900 \text{ minutes}}$

   $= 16.666 \text{ gtt/min}$

   $= 17 \text{ gtt/min}$

6. $60 \text{ minutes} = 1 \text{ hour}$

   $X \text{ gtt/min} = \dfrac{60 \text{ mL} \times 10 \text{ gtt/mL}}{60 \text{ minutes}}$

   $X \text{ gtt/min} = \dfrac{600 \text{ gtt}}{60 \text{ minutes}}$

   $= 10 \text{ gtt/min}$

7. $360 \text{ minutes} = 6 \text{ hours} \times 60 \text{ minutes}$

   $X \text{ gtt/min} = \dfrac{500 \text{ mL} \times 10 \text{ gtt/mL}}{360 \text{ minutes}}$

   $X \text{ gtt/min} = \dfrac{5000 \text{ gtt}}{360 \text{ minutes}}$

   $= 13.888 \text{ gtt/min}$

   $= 14 \text{ gtt/min}$

8. $X \text{ gtt/min} = \dfrac{25 \text{ mL} \times 15 \text{ gtt/mL}}{30 \text{ minutes}}$

   $X \text{ gtt/min} = \dfrac{375 \text{ gtt}}{30 \text{ minutes}}$

   $= 12.5 \text{ gtt/min}$

   $= 13 \text{ gtt/min}$

9. 300 minutes = 5 hours × 60 minutes

$$X \text{ gtt/min} = \frac{1000 \text{ mL} \times 15 \text{ gtt/mL}}{300 \text{ minutes}}$$

$$X \text{ gtt/min} = \frac{15,000 \text{ gtt}}{300 \text{ minutes}}$$

$$= 50 \text{ gtt/min}$$

10. 1440 minutes = 24 hours × 60 minutes

$$X \text{ gtt/min} = \frac{2000 \text{ mL} \times 10 \text{ gtt/mL}}{1440 \text{ minutes}}$$

$$X \text{ gtt/min} = \frac{20,000 \text{ gtt}}{1440 \text{ minutes}}$$

$$= 13.888 \text{ gtt/min}$$

$$= 14 \text{ gtt/min}$$

CASE STUDY

CASE 2

Calculate the pump settings for the following orders.

QUESTION 1. Medication order: 1000 mL D5W I.V. over 24 hours
What is the pump setting?

QUESTION 2. Medication order: 200 mL Lactated Ringers I.V. over 5 hours
What is the pump setting?

QUESTION 3. Medication order: 1500 mL normal saline I.V. over 12 hours
What is the pump setting?

QUESTION 4. Medication order: 500 mL D5 1/2 normal saline I.V. over 8 hours
What is the pump setting?

QUESTION 5. Medication order: 800 mL ½ normal saline I.V. over 16 hours
What is the pump setting?

QUESTION 6. Medication order: 50 mL D5 normal saline I.V. over 1 hour
What is the pump setting?

QUESTION 7. Medication order: 350 mL D5W I.V. over 4 hours
What is the pump setting?

QUESTION 8. Medication order: 3000 mL normal saline I.V. over 24 hours
What is the pump setting?

QUESTION 9. Medication order: 1500 mL Lactated Ringers I.V. over 16 hours
What is the pump setting?

QUESTION 10. Medication order: 150 mL D5 1/2 normal saline I.V. over 5 hours
What is the pump setting?

ANSWERS

1. $mL/hr = \dfrac{1000 \text{ mL}}{24 \text{ hours}}$

   $mL/hr = 41.666 \text{ mL}$

   $mL/hr = 42 \text{ mL}$

2. $mL/hr = \dfrac{200 \text{ mL}}{5 \text{ hours}}$

   $mL/hr = 40 \text{ mL}$

3. $mL/hr = \dfrac{1500 \text{ mL}}{12 \text{ hours}}$

   $mL/hr = 125 \text{ mL}$

4. $mL/hr = \dfrac{500 \text{ mL}}{8 \text{ hours}}$

   $mL/hr = 62.5 \text{ mL}$

   $mL/hr = 63 \text{ mL}$

5. $mL/hr = \dfrac{800 \text{ mL}}{6 \text{ hours}}$

   $133.33 = 133 \text{ mL}$

6. $mL/hr = \dfrac{50 \text{ mL}}{1 \text{ hour}}$

   $mL/hr = 50 \text{ mL}$

7. $mL/hr = \dfrac{350 \text{ mL}}{4 \text{ hours}}$

   $mL/hr = 87.5 \text{ mL}$

   $mL/hr = 88 \text{ mL}$

8. $mL/hr = \dfrac{3000 \text{ mL}}{24 \text{ hours}}$

   $mL/hr = 125$ mL

9. $mL/hr = \dfrac{1500 \text{ mL}}{16 \text{ hours}}$

   $mL/hr = 93.75$ mL

   $mL/hr = 94$ mL

10. $mL/hr = \dfrac{150 \text{ mL}}{5 \text{ hours}}$

   $mL/hr = 30$ mL

CASE STUDY

CASE 3

Calculate the remaining infusion time for the following patients. Assume that the I.V. bag contains the total amount that is being infused.

QUESTION 1. 1000 mL D5W I.V. The pump setting is 42 mL. Current volume in the I.V. bag is 750 mL.
How much time is remaining?

QUESTION 2. 200 mL Lactated Ringers I.V. The pump setting is 40 mL. Current volume in the I.V. bag is 150 mL.
How much time is remaining?

QUESTION 3. 1500 mL normal saline I.V. The pump setting is 125 mL. Current volume in the I.V. bag is 500 mL.
How much time is remaining?

QUESTION 4. 500 mL D5 1/2 normal saline I.V. The pump setting is 63 mL. Current volume in the I.V. bag is 200 mL.
How much time is remaining?

QUESTION 5. 800 mL ½ normal saline I.V. The pump setting is 50 mL. Current volume in the I.V. bag is 300 mL.
How much time is remaining?

QUESTION 6. 50 mL D5 normal saline I.V. The pump setting is 50 mL. Current volume in the I.V. bag is 25 mL.
How much time is remaining?

QUESTION 7. 350 mL D5W I.V. The pump setting is 88 mL. Current volume in the I.V. bag is 150 mL.
How much time is remaining?

QUESTION 8. 3000 mL normal saline I.V. The pump setting is 125 mL. Current volume in the I.V. bag is 2500 mL.
How much time is remaining?

QUESTION 9. 1500 mL Lactated Ringers I.V. The pump setting is 94 mL. Current volume in the I.V. bag is 500 mL.
How much time is remaining?

QUESTION 10. 150 mL D51/2 normal saline I.V. The pump setting is 30 mL. Current volume in the I.V. bag is 25 mL.
How much time is remaining?

ANSWERS

1. Time remaining $= \dfrac{750 \text{ mL}}{42 \text{ mL}}$

   Time remaining $= 17.86$ hours

   Minutes $= 60$ minutes $\times 0.86 = 51.6$ minutes

   Time remaining $= 17$ hours 52 minutes

2. Time remaining $= \dfrac{150 \text{ mL}}{40 \text{ mL}}$

   Time remaining $= 3.75$ hours

   Minutes $= 60$ minutes $\times 0.75 = 45$ minutes

   Time remaining $= 3$ hours 45 minutes

3. Time remaining $= \dfrac{500 \text{ mL}}{125 \text{ mL}}$

   Time remaining $= 4$ hours

4. Time remaining $= \dfrac{200 \text{ mL}}{63 \text{ mL}}$

   Time remaining $= 3.17$ hrs

   Minutes $= 60$ minutes $\times 0.17 = 10$ minutes

   Time remaining $= 3$ hours 10 minutes

5. Time remaining $= \dfrac{300 \text{ mL}}{50 \text{ mL}}$

   Time remaining $= 6$ hours

6. Time remaining $= \dfrac{25 \text{ mL}}{50 \text{ mL}}$

   Time remaining $= 0.5$ hours

   Minutes $= 60$ minutes $\times 0.5 = 30$ minutes

   Time remaining $= 30$ minutes

7. Time remaining $= \dfrac{150 \text{ mL}}{88 \text{ mL}}$

   Time remaining $= 1.70$ hours

   Minutes $= 60$ minutes $\times 0.70 = 42$ minutes

   Time remaining $= 1$ hour 42 minutes

8. Time remaining $= \dfrac{2500 \text{ mL}}{125 \text{ mL}}$

   Time remaining $= 20$ hours

9. Time remaining $= \dfrac{500 \text{ mL}}{94 \text{ mL}}$

   Time remaining $= 5.31$ hours

   Minutes $= 60$ minutes $\times 0.31 = 19$ minutes

   Time remaining $= 5$ hours 19 minutes

10. Time remaining $= \dfrac{25 \text{ mL}}{30 \text{ mL}}$

    Time remaining $= 0.83$ hours

    Minutes $= 60$ minutes $\times 0.83 = 49.8$ minutes

    Time remaining $= 50$ minutes

FINAL CHECK-UP

1. The medication order is for 1000 mL of D5W I.V. that is to be administered over 5 hours. What is the pump setting?

   A. 2 mL

   B. 200 mL

   C. 20 mL

   D. 0.2 mL

2. The medication order is for 1 L of normal saline I.V. that is to be administered over 8 hours. On hand is I.V. tubing with a 10 gtt/mL drip factor. What is the drip setting?

   A. 21 gtt/min
   B. 2.1 gtt/min
   C. 210 gtt/min
   D. 20 gtt/min

3. The medication order is for Cefadyl 10 g diluted in 200 mL of normal saline I.V. that is to be administered over 4 hours. On hand is I.V. tubing with a 15 gtt/mL drip factor. What is the drip setting?

   A. 12 gtt/min
   B. 12.5 gtt/min
   C. 13 gtt/min
   D. 13.5 gtt/min

4. The medication order is for 200 mL of D5W I.V. that is to be administered over 4 hours. The nurse should set the pump at 50 mL/hr.

   A. True
   B. False

5. Your patient has received 250 mL of normal saline I.V. and the I.V. bag currently has a volume of 75 mL of normal saline. The pump is set at 30 mL/hr. How much longer does the infusion have to run?

   A. 2 hours 35 minutes
   B. 30 minutes
   C. 2 hours
   D. 2 hours 30 minutes

6. The medication order is for 200 mL of D5 1/2 normal saline I.V. that is to be administered over 7 hours. On hand is I.V. tubing with a 10 gtt/mL drip factor. What is the drip setting?

   A. 5 gtt/min
   B. 5.5 gtt/min
   C. 4 gtt/min
   D. 4.8 gtt/min

7. The medication order is for 3000 mL of ½ normal saline I.V. that is to be administered over 24 hours. What is the pump setting?

   A. 124 mL/hr
   B. 120 mL/hr
   C. 125 mL/hr
   D. 126 mL/hr

8. The medication order is for 2000 mL of Ringers Lactate I.V. that is to be administered over 16 hours. On hand is I.V. tubing with a 15 gtt/mL drip factor. What is the drip setting?

   A. 31 gtt/min
   B. 31.5 gtt/min
   C. 32 gtt/min
   D. 32.5 gtt/min

9. The medication order is for 600 mL of ½ normal saline I.V. that is to be administered over 6 hours. On hand is I.V. tubing with a 10 gtt/mL drip factor. What is the pump setting?

   A. 100 mL/hr
   B. 90 mL/hr
   C. 80 mL/hr
   D. 110 mL/hr

10. Your patient has received 1500 mL of normal saline I.V. and the I.V. bag currently has a volume of 750 mL of normal saline. The pump is set at 40 mL/hr. How much longer does the infusion have to run?

   A. 18 hours 35 minutes
   B. 10 hours 45 minutes
   C. 8 hours 45 minutes
   D. 18 hours 45 minutes

CORRECT ANSWERS AND RATIONALES

1. B. 200 mL
2. A. 21 gtt/min
3. C. 13 gtt/min
4. A. True
5. D. 2 hours 30 minutes
6. D. 4.8 gtt/min
7. C. 125 mL/hr
8. A. 31 gtt/min
9. A. 100 mL/hr
10. D. 18 hours 45 minutes

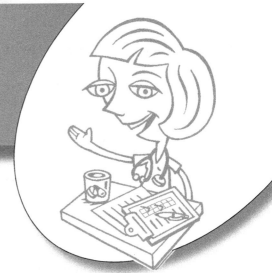

chapter **5**

Calculating Pediatric Doses

LEARNING OBJECTIVES

1. Calculating Pediatric Doses
2. The Pediatric Dose Calculation Formula
3. Calculating the Maximum Quantity per Day
4. Calculating Multiple Doses

> ## KEY TERMS
>
> Calculating Using the Multiple Dose Formula
>
> Calculating Using the Pediatric Dose Formula
>
> From Pounds to Kilogram
>
> Rounding
>
> The Multiple Dose Formula

You were taught in school that pediatric patients are not simply small versions of adult patients. Instead, pediatric patients are at various states of maturity and may lack the capability to adequately metabolize and excrete medications at an adult dose.

The dose of medication for a pediatric patient must be carefully calculated based on the patient's weight because even a small discrepancy can endanger the youngster's health. Furthermore, there is a limit on the amount of a medication that the pediatric patient can receive within 24 hours.

Before administering medication, you'll need to determine the total amount of the medication the youngster has already received and then calculate the dose using the patient's weight. You'll learn how to perform both calculations in this chapter.

1. Calculating Pediatric Doses

The dose of a medication prescribed for an adult is based on a typical adult. The physician may adjust the dose if the patient's condition differs from that of a typical adult because of age or condition of the patient's body. For example, the dose may be decreased for elderly patients or patients with liver disease since the medication is absorbed and metabolized slower than in a typical adult.

In contrast, pediatric medication is prescribed in a dose that is relatively unique for the patient because the prescribed dose is based on the child's weight. The quantity of the medication is written in the medication order per kilogram.

Here's an example:

Elixir of Digoxin 15 mcg

From Pounds to Kilogram

Although some health care facilities may record a patient's weight in kilogram, many record the patient's weight in pounds. You'll need to convert the child's weight from pounds to kilograms before calculating the dose.

The conversion process is straightforward if you remember that
1 kg = 2.2 lb
Then use the following formula for the conversion.

$$\text{Child's weight (kg)} = \frac{\text{child's weight (lb)}}{2.2 \text{ lb}}$$

Let's say that child weighs 66 lb and you need to convert this weight to kilograms. Here's what to do:

1. Insert values into the formula.

$$\text{Child's weight (kg)} = \frac{66 \text{ lb}}{2.2 \text{ lb}}$$

2. Calculate the formula.

$$30 \text{ kg} = \frac{66 \text{ lb}}{2.2 \text{ lb}}$$

Rounding

Expect decimal values when you convert from pounds to kilograms. This isn't a problem as long as you apply the rounding rules that you learned in Chapter 2. Here's what to do:

1. Truncate the kilogram weight to three decimal values.

2. Don't round the kilogram weight.

3. Use the kilogram weight—and its three decimal values—in the pediatric dose calculation.

Suppose the child weighs 50 lb. Insert this value into the formula and calculate. This results in a series of decimal values of 7272727…. Use three decimal values only as shown here:

$$22.727 \text{ kg} = \frac{50 \text{ lb}}{2.2 \text{ lb}}$$

NURSING ALERT

It is always a good practice to ask another registered nurse to double check your calculations as a precaution.

2. The Pediatric Dose Calculation Formula

The pediatric dose calculation formula is very similar to the formula used to calculate an adult dose (see Chapter 2) except the quantity of medication ordered is for 1 kg of the patient's weight. You must first determine the full quantity ordered for the patient and then the dose to administer to the patient.

There are four components of the pediatric dose calculation formula as shown here:

$$\text{Dose} = \frac{\text{orders per kg} \times \text{patient's weight (kg)}}{\text{Dose on hand}} \times \text{quantity on hand}$$

Calculating Using the Pediatric Dose Formula

Let's calculate the dose for Elixir of Digoxin 15 mcg/kg. The patient weighs 66 lb. Previously in this chapter ("From Pounds to Kilogram") the patient's weight was converted to 30 kg. The medication label reads 50 mcg/mL.

1. Insert values into the formula.

$$\text{Dose} = \frac{15 \text{ mcg/kg} \times 30 \text{ kg}}{50 \text{ mcg}} \times 1 \text{ mL}$$

2. Calculate the full quantity ordered by multiplying the quantity per kilogram by the patient's weight.

$$\text{Dose} = \frac{450 \text{ mcg}}{50 \text{ mcg}} \times 1 \text{ mL}$$

3. Calculate the dose as you would calculate an adult dose (see Chapter 2).

$$\text{Dose} = 9 \text{ mcg} \times 1 \text{ mL}$$
$$\text{Dose} = 9 \text{ mcg}$$

3. Calculating the Maximum Quantity per Day

Drug manufacturers determine the maximum quantity of a medication that a child can receive within a 24-hour period. A medication order that exceeds the allowable amount must be questioned because the physician may not be aware of the amount of the medication that the child has already received.

Before administering medication to the child, you must determine the maximum quantity of the medication that is permissible within a 24-hour period. You'll find this information in a drug guide on the unit.

Next, review the Medication Administration Record (see Chapter 1) and calculate the total amount of the medication that the child received within the last 24 hours.

Next, calculate the dose you plan to administer to the child. Add this amount to the total the child received so far within 24 hours and compare the result to the maximum allowable from the drug guide.

If child hasn't received the maximum amount, then administer the next dose, otherwise don't administer the medication. Report your findings to the physician.

4. Calculating Multiple Doses

Typically the patient receives multiple doses of the same medication over course of a day. The physician may order a loading dose first followed by a series of maintenance doses. The loading dose is a high dose to deliver a larger amount of medication to the patient quickly. A maintenance dose is a lower dose designed to maintain the therapeutic level of the medication.

The medication order for the maintenance doses usually specifies a daily quantity of medication that is to be administered multiple times during the day. For example, the physician might write

Ampicillin 50 mg/kg per day q6h

You need to calculate the dose that is to be administered every 6 hours.

The Multiple Dose Formula

The multiple dose formula is very similar to the pediatric dose calculation formula. Both formulas result in a dose; however, the multiple dose formula results in the dose for the entire 24-hour period and therefore must be divided by the number of doses specified in the medication order.

Here is the multiple dose formula:

$$\text{Dose/day} = \frac{\text{orders/kg} \times \text{patient's weight (kg)}}{\text{on hand}} \times \text{quantity on hand}$$

$$\text{Dose} = \frac{\text{dose/day}}{\text{ordered number of doses}}$$

Calculating Using the Multiple Dose Formula

Let's calculate the dose for Ampicillin 50 mg/kg · day every 6 hours. The patient weighs 30 lb. Previously in this chapter ("From Pounds to Kilogram") the patient's weight was converted to 13.636 kg. The medication label reads 100 mg/mL.

1. Insert values into the formula.

$$\text{Dose per day} = \frac{50 \text{ mg} \times 13.636 \text{ kg}}{100 \text{ mg}} \times 1 \text{ mL}$$

2. Calculate the **dose per day**.

$$\text{Dose per day} = \frac{50 \text{ mg} \times 13.636 \text{ kg}}{100 \text{ mg}} \times 1 \text{ mL}$$

$$\text{Dose per day} = \frac{681.8 \text{ mg}}{100 \text{ mg}} \times 1 \text{ mL}$$

$$\text{Dose per day} = 6.818 \text{ mg} \times 1 \text{ mL}$$

$$\text{Dose per day} = 6.8 \text{ mL}$$

3. Insert values into the formula.

$$\text{Dose} = \frac{6.8 \text{ mL}}{4 \text{ doses ordered}}$$

4. Calculate the dose.

$$\text{Dose} = 1.7 \text{ mL}$$

NURSING ALERT

Table 1–3 in Chapter 1 contains abbreviations used to specify the frequency to administer a medication to a patient. If order specifies the frequency in hours such as every 6 hours (q6h), divide 24 hours by the frequency to identify the number of doses that must be administered to the patient. For example,

---

$$4 \text{ doses} = \frac{24 \text{ hours}}{6}$$

CASE STUDY

CASE 1

Calculate the correct dose using the pediatric dose calculation formula for the following orders.

QUESTION 1. Medication order: Benadryl 10 mg/kg
The patient weighs 26 lb.
Medication label: Benadryl 125 mg/5 mL
How many milliliters will be administered to the patient?

QUESTION 2. Medication order: Benylin 5 mg/kg
The patient weighs 44 lb.
Medication label: Benylin 50 mg per tablet
How many tablets will be administered to the patient?

QUESTION 3. Medication order: Lithostat 15 mg/kg
The patient weighs 70 lb.
Medication label: Lithostat 250 mg per tablet
How many tablets will be administered to the patient?

QUESTION 4. Medication order: Zovirax 5 mg/kg
The patient weighs 30 lb.
Medication label: Zovirax 25 mg/mL
How many milliliters will be administered to the patient?

QUESTION 5. Medication order: Ampicillin 12.5 mg/kg
The patient weighs 40 lb.
Medication label: Ampicillin 100 mg/mL
How many milliliters will be administered to the patient?

QUESTION 6. Medication order: Zofran 150 mcg/kg
The patient weighs 65 lb.
Medication label: Zofran 2000 mcg/mL
How many milliliters will be administered to the patient?

QUESTION 7. Medication order: Dilantin 1 mg/kg
The patient weighs 66 lb.
Medication label: Dilantin 15 mg/capsule
How many milliliters will be administered to the patient?

QUESTION 8. Medication order: Amoxicillin 10 mg/kg
The patient weighs 30 lb.
Medication label: Amoxicillin 125 mg/5 mL
How many milliliters will be administered to the patient?

QUESTION 9. Medication order: Celocin 6.25 mg/kg
The patient weighs 45 lb.
Medication label: Celocin 75 mg/5 mL
How many milliliters will be administered to the patient?

QUESTION 10. Medication order: Cephalexin 15 mg/kg
The patient weighs 45 lb.
Medication label: Cephalexin 125 mg/5 mL
How many milliliters will be administered to the patient?

ANSWERS

1. $11.818 \text{ kg} = \dfrac{26 \text{ lb}}{2.2 \text{ lb}}$

$$\text{Dose} = \dfrac{10 \text{ mg} \times 11.818 \text{ kg}}{125 \text{ mg}} \times 5 \text{ mL}$$

$$\text{Dose} = \dfrac{118.18 \text{ mg}}{125 \text{ mg}} \times 5 \text{ mL}$$

$$\text{Dose} = 0.945 \times 5 \text{ mL}$$

$$\text{Dose} = 4.727 \text{ mL}$$

$$\text{Dose} = 4.7 \text{ mL}$$

2. $20 \text{ kg} = \dfrac{44 \text{ lb}}{2.2 \text{ lb}}$

$$\text{Dose} = \dfrac{5 \text{ mg} \times 20 \text{ kg}}{50 \text{ mg}} \times 1 \text{ tablet}$$

$$\text{Dose} = \dfrac{100 \text{ mg}}{50 \text{ mg}} \times 1 \text{ tablet}$$

$$\text{Dose} = 2 \times 1 \text{ tablet}$$

$$\text{Dose} = 2 \text{ tablets}$$

3. $31.818 \, \text{kg} = \dfrac{70 \, \text{lb}}{2.2 \, \text{lb}}$

$\text{Dose} = \dfrac{15 \, \text{mg} \times 31.818 \, \text{kg}}{250 \, \text{mg}} \times 1 \, \text{tablet}$

$\text{Dose} = \dfrac{477.27 \, \text{mg}}{250 \, \text{mg}} \times 1 \, \text{tablet}$

$\text{Dose} = 1.909 \, \text{mg}$

$\text{Dose} = 1.909 \times 1 \, \text{tablet}$

$\text{Dose} = 2 \, \text{tablets}$

4. $13.636 \, \text{kg} = \dfrac{30 \, \text{lb}}{2.2 \, \text{lb}}$

$\text{Dose} = \dfrac{5 \, \text{mg} \times 13.636 \, \text{kg}}{25 \, \text{mg}} \times 1 \, \text{mL}$

$\text{Dose} = \dfrac{68.18 \, \text{mg}}{25 \, \text{mg}} \times 1 \, \text{mL}$

$\text{Dose} = 2.727 \, \text{mg}$

$\text{Dose} = 2.727 \, \text{mg} \times 1 \, \text{mL}$

$\text{Dose} = 2.7 \, \text{mL}$

5. $18.181 \, \text{kg} = \dfrac{40 \, \text{lb}}{2.2 \, \text{lb}}$

$\text{Dose} = \dfrac{12.5 \, \text{mg} \times 18.181 \, \text{kg}}{100 \, \text{mg}} \times 1 \, \text{mL}$

$\text{Dose} = \dfrac{227.262 \, \text{mg}}{100 \, \text{mg}} \times 1 \, \text{mL}$

$\text{Dose} = 2.272 \, \text{mg}$

$\text{Dose} = 2.272 \, \text{mg} \times 1 \, \text{mL}$

$\text{Dose} = 2.3 \, \text{mL}$

6. $29.545 \, \text{kg} = \dfrac{65 \, \text{lb}}{2.2 \, \text{lb}}$

$\text{Dose} = \dfrac{150 \, \text{mcg} \times 29.545 \, \text{kg}}{2000 \, \text{mcg}} \times 1 \, \text{mL}$

$\text{Dose} = \dfrac{4431.75 \, \text{mcg}}{2000 \, \text{mcg}} \times 1 \, \text{mL}$

$\text{Dose} = 2.215 \, \text{mcg}$

$\text{Dose} = 2.215 \, \text{mcg} \times 1 \, \text{mL}$

$\text{Dose} = 2.2 \, \text{mL}$

7. $30 \, \text{kg} = \dfrac{66 \, \text{lb}}{2.2 \, \text{lb}}$

$\text{Dose} = \dfrac{1 \, \text{mg} \times 30 \, \text{kg}}{15 \, \text{mg}} \times 1 \, \text{capsule}$

$\text{Dose} = \dfrac{30 \, \text{mg}}{15 \, \text{mg}} \times 1 \, \text{capsule}$

$\text{Dose} = 2 \, \text{mg} \times 1 \, \text{capsule}$

$\text{Dose} = 2 \, \text{capsules}$

8. $13.636 \, \text{kg} = \dfrac{30 \, \text{lb}}{2.2 \, \text{lb}}$

$\text{Dose} = \dfrac{10 \, \text{mg} \times 13.636 \, \text{kg}}{125 \, \text{mg}} \times 5 \, \text{mL}$

$\text{Dose} = \dfrac{136.36 \, \text{mg}}{125 \, \text{mg}} \times 5 \, \text{mL}$

$\text{Dose} = 1.090 \, \text{mg} \times 5 \, \text{mL}$

$\text{Dose} = 5.454 \, \text{mL}$

$\text{Dose} = 5.5 \, \text{mL}$

9. $20.454 \, \text{kg} = \dfrac{45 \, \text{lb}}{2.2 \, \text{lb}}$

$\text{Dose} = \dfrac{6.25 \, \text{mg} \times 20.454 \, \text{kg}}{75 \, \text{mg}} \times 5 \, \text{mL}$

$\text{Dose} = \dfrac{127.837 \, \text{mg}}{75 \, \text{mg}} \times 5 \, \text{mL}$

$\text{Dose} = 1.704 \, \text{mg} \times 5 \, \text{mL}$

$\text{Dose} = 8.522 \, \text{mL}$

$\text{Dose} = 8.5 \, \text{mL}$

10. $20.454 \, \text{kg} = \dfrac{45 \, \text{lb}}{2.2 \, \text{lb}}$

$\text{Dose} = \dfrac{15 \, \text{mg} \times 20.454 \, \text{kg}}{125 \, \text{mg}} \times 5 \, \text{mL}$

$\text{Dose} = \dfrac{306.81 \, \text{mg}}{125 \, \text{mg}} \times 5 \, \text{mL}$

$\text{Dose} = 2.454 \, \text{mg} \times 5 \, \text{mL}$

$\text{Dose} = 12.274 \, \text{mL}$

$\text{Dose} = 12 \, \text{mL}$

CASE STUDY

CASE 2
Calculate the correct dose using the multidose calculation formula for the following orders.

QUESTION 1. Medication order: Benadryl 30 mg/kg/day q6h
The patient weighs 66 lb.
Medication label: Benadryl 125 mg/5 mL
How many milliliters per dose will be administered to the patient?

QUESTION 2. Medication order: Benylin 25 mg/kg/day q3h
The patient weighs 55 lb.
Medication label: Benylin 25 mg/mL
How many milliliters per dose will be administered to the patient?

QUESTION 3. Medication order: Lithostat 120 mg/kg/day q4h
The patient weighs 110 lb.
Medication label: Lithostat 250 mg/mL
How many milliliters per dose will be administered to the patient?

QUESTION 4. Medication order: Zovirax 5 mg/kg/day q12h
The patient weighs 55 lb.
Medication label: Zovirax 25 mg per tablet
How many tablets per dose will be administered to the patient?

QUESTION 5. Medication order: Ampicillin 15 mg/kg/day q8/h
The patient weighs 44 lb.
Medication label: Ampicillin 100 mg/mL
How many milliliters per dose will be administered to the patient?

QUESTION 6. Medication order: Zofran 120 mg/kg/day q6h
The patient weighs 33 lb.
Medication label: Zofran 200 mg/mL
How many milliliters per dose will be administered to the patient?

QUESTION 7. Medication order: Dilantin 30 mg/kg/day q8h
The patient weighs 55 lb.
Medication label: Dilantin 40 mg/mL
How many milliliters per dose will be administered to the patient?

QUESTION 8. Medication order: Amoxicillin 10 mg/kg/day q6h
The patient weighs 44 lb.
Medication label: Amoxicillin 125 mg/5 mL
How many milliliters per dose will be administered to the patient?

QUESTION 9. Medication order: Celocin 45 mg/kg/day q4h
The patient weighs 110 lb.
Medication label: Celocin 125 mg/5 mL
How many milliliters per dose will be administered to the patient?

QUESTION 10. Medication order: Cephalexin 15 mg/kg/day q6h
The patient weighs 132 lb.
Medication label: Cephalexin 125 mg/5 mL
How many milliliters per dose will be administered to the patient?

ANSWERS

1. $4 \text{ doses} = \dfrac{24 \text{ hours}}{6}$

   $30 \text{ kg} = \dfrac{66 \text{ lb}}{2.2 \text{ lb}}$

   $\text{Dose per day} = \dfrac{30 \text{ mg} \times 30 \text{ kg}}{125 \text{ mg}} \times 5 \text{ mL}$

   $\phantom{\text{Dose per day}} = \dfrac{900 \text{ mg}}{125 \text{ mg}} \times 5 \text{ mL}$

   $\text{Dose per day} = 7.2 \text{ mg} \times 5 \text{ mL}$

   $\text{Dose per day} = 36 \text{ mL}$

   $\text{Per dose} = \dfrac{36 \text{ mL}}{4 \text{ doses}}$

   $\text{Per dose} = 9 \text{ mL}$

2. $$8 \text{ doses} = \frac{24 \text{ hours}}{3}$$

$$25 \text{ kg} = \frac{55 \text{ lb}}{2.2 \text{ lb}}$$

$$\text{Dose per day} = \frac{50 \text{ mg} \times 25 \text{ kg}}{25 \text{ mg}} \times 1 \text{ mL}$$

$$= \frac{1250 \text{ mg}}{25 \text{ mg}} \times 1 \text{ mL}$$

$$\text{Dose per day} = 50 \text{ mg} \times 1 \text{ mL}$$

$$\text{Dose per day} = 50 \text{ mL}$$

$$\text{Per dose} = \frac{50 \text{ mL}}{8 \text{ doses}}$$

$$\text{Per dose} = 6.25 \text{ mL}$$

3. $$6 \text{ doses} = \frac{24 \text{ hours}}{4}$$

$$50 \text{ kg} = \frac{110 \text{ lb}}{2.2 \text{ lb}}$$

$$\text{Dose per day} = \frac{120 \text{ mg} \times 50 \text{ kg}}{250 \text{ mg}} \times 1 \text{ mL}$$

$$= \frac{6000 \text{ mg}}{250 \text{ mg}} \times 1 \text{ mL}$$

$$\text{Dose per day} = 24 \text{ mg} \times 1 \text{ mL}$$

$$\text{Dose per day} = 24 \text{ mL}$$

$$\text{Per dose} = \frac{24 \text{ mL}}{6 \text{ doses}}$$

$$\text{Per dose} = 4 \text{ mL}$$

4. $$2 \text{ doses} = \frac{24 \text{ hours}}{12}$$

$$25 \text{ kg} = \frac{55 \text{ lb}}{2.2 \text{ lb}}$$

$$\text{Dose per day} = \frac{5 \text{ mg} \times 25 \text{ kg}}{25 \text{ mg}} \times 1 \text{ tablet}$$

$$= \frac{125 \text{ mg}}{25 \text{ mg}} \times 1 \text{ tablet}$$

$$\text{Dose per day} = 5 \text{ mg} \times 1 \text{ tablet}$$

$$\text{Dose per day} = 5 \text{ tablets}$$

$$\text{Per dose} = \frac{5 \text{ tablets}}{2 \text{ doses}}$$

$$\text{Per dose} = 2.5 \text{ tablets}$$

5. $3 \text{ doses} = \dfrac{24 \text{ hours}}{8}$

$20 \text{ kg} = \dfrac{44 \text{ lb}}{2.2 \text{ lb}}$

$\text{Dose per day} = \dfrac{15 \text{ mg} \times 20 \text{ kg}}{100 \text{ mg}} \times 1 \text{ mL}$

$= \dfrac{300 \text{ mg}}{100 \text{ mg}} \times 1 \text{ mL}$

$\text{Dose per day} = 3 \text{ mg} \times 1 \text{ mL}$

$\text{Dose per day} = 3 \text{ mL}$

$\text{Per dose} = \dfrac{3 \text{ mL}}{3 \text{ doses}}$

$\text{Per dose} = 1 \text{ mL}$

6. $4 \text{ doses} = \dfrac{24 \text{ hours}}{6}$

$15 \text{ kg} = \dfrac{33 \text{ lb}}{2.2 \text{ lb}}$

$\text{Dose per day} = \dfrac{120 \text{ mg} \times 15 \text{ kg}}{200 \text{ mg}} \times 1 \text{ mL}$

$= \dfrac{1800 \text{ mg}}{200 \text{ mg}} \times 1 \text{ mL}$

$\text{Dose per day} = 9 \text{ mg} \times 1 \text{ mL}$

$\text{Dose per day} = 9 \text{ mL}$

$\text{Per dose} = \dfrac{9 \text{ mL}}{4 \text{ doses}}$

$\text{Per dose} = 2.25 \text{ mL}$

7. $3 \text{ doses} = \dfrac{24 \text{ hours}}{8}$

$25 \text{ kg} = \dfrac{55 \text{ lb}}{2.2 \text{ lb}}$

$\text{Dose per day} = \dfrac{30 \text{ mg} \times 25 \text{ kg}}{40 \text{ mg}} \times 1 \text{ mL}$

$= \dfrac{750 \text{ mg}}{40 \text{ mg}} \times 1 \text{ mL}$

$\text{Dose per day} = 18.75 \text{ mg} \times 1 \text{ mL}$

$\text{Dose per day} = 18.75 \text{ mL}$

$\text{Per dose} = \dfrac{18.75 \text{ mL}}{3 \text{ doses}}$

$\text{Per dose} = 6.25 \text{ mL}$

8. $4 \text{ doses} = \dfrac{24 \text{ hours}}{6}$

$20 \text{ kg} = \dfrac{44 \text{ lb}}{2.2 \text{ lb}}$

$\text{Dose per day} = \dfrac{10 \text{ mg} \times 20 \text{ kg}}{125 \text{ mg}} \times 5 \text{ mL}$

$= \dfrac{200 \text{ mg}}{125 \text{ mg}} \times 5 \text{ mL}$

$\text{Dose per day} = 1.6 \text{ mg} \times 5 \text{ mL}$

$\text{Dose per day} = 8 \text{ mL}$

$\text{Per dose} = \dfrac{8 \text{ mL}}{4 \text{ doses}}$

$\text{Per dose} = 2 \text{ mL}$

9. $6 \text{ doses} = \dfrac{24 \text{ hours}}{4}$

$50 \text{ kg} = \dfrac{110 \text{ lb}}{2.2 \text{ lb}}$

$\text{Dose per day} = \dfrac{45 \text{ mg} \times 50 \text{ kg}}{125 \text{ mg}} \times 5 \text{ mL}$

$= \dfrac{2250 \text{ mg}}{125 \text{ mg}} \times 5 \text{ mL}$

$\text{Dose per day} = 18 \text{ mg} \times 5 \text{ mL}$

$\text{Dose per day} = 90 \text{ mL}$

$\text{Per dose} = \dfrac{90 \text{ mL}}{6 \text{ doses}}$

$\text{Per dose} = 15 \text{ mL}$

10. $4 \text{ doses} = \dfrac{24 \text{ hours}}{6}$

$60 \text{ kg} = \dfrac{132 \text{ lb}}{2.2 \text{ lb}}$

$\text{Dose per day} = \dfrac{15 \text{ mg} \times 60 \text{ kg}}{125 \text{ mg}} \times 5 \text{ mL}$

$= \dfrac{900 \text{ mg}}{125 \text{ mg}} \times 5 \text{ mL}$

$\text{Dose per day} = 7.2 \text{ mg} \times 5 \text{ mL}$

$\text{Dose per day} = 36 \text{ mL}$

$\text{Per dose} = \dfrac{36 \text{ mL}}{4 \text{ doses}}$

$\text{Per dose} = 9 \text{ mL}$

FINAL CHECK-UP

1. The physician ordered Digoxin 15 mcg/kg. The patient weighs 44 lb. The medication label reads 75 mcg/mL. What dose will you administer to the patient?

   A. 4 mL

   B. 400 mL

   C. 40 mL

   D. 0.4 mL

2. The physician ordered Dilantin 45 mg/kg · day q4h. The patient weighs 110 lb. The medication label reads 125 mg/5 mL. What dose will you administer to the patient?

   A. 21 mL

   B. 1.5 mL

   C. 15 mL

   D. 20 mL

3. The physician ordered Ampicillin 5 mg/kg. The patient weighs 55 lb. The medication label reads 25 mg/mL. What dose will you administer to the patient?

   A. 0.5 mL

   B. 5 mL

   C. 50 mL

   D. 0.05 mL

4. The physician ordered Zofran 120 mg/kg. The patient weighs 33 lb. The medication label reads 200 mg/mL. You will administer 9 mL to the patient.

   A. True

   B. False

5. The physician ordered Lithostat 15 mg/kg. The patient weighs 44 lb. The medication label reads 100 mg/mL. What dose will you administer to the patient?

   A. 5 mL

   B. 4 mL

   C. 3 mL

   D. 2 mL

6. The physician ordered Celocin 10 mg/kg · day q6h. The patient weighs 44 lb. The medication label reads 125 mg/mL. What dose will you administer to the patient?

   A. 0.5 mL

   B. 0.2 mL

   C. 0.4 mL

   D. 0.3 mL

7. The physician ordered Benylin 120 mg/kg. The patient weighs 33 lb. The medication label reads 200 mg/mL. What dose will you administer to the patient?

   A. 1 mL
   B. 1.9 mL
   C. 0.9 mL
   D. 9 mL

8. The physician ordered Benadryl 15 mg/kg. The patient weighs 132 lb. The medication label reads 125 mg/mL. What dose will you administer to the patient?

   A. 7.2 mL
   B. 7 mL
   C. 8 mL
   D. 0.72 mL

9. The physician ordered Ampicillin 30 mg/kg. The patient weighs 22 lb. The medication label reads 125 mg/mL. What dose will you administer to the patient?

   A. 2 mL
   B. 0.24 mL
   C. 24 mL
   D. 2.4 mL

10. The physician ordered Zovirax 10 mg/kg. The patient weighs 77 lb. The medication label reads 100 mg/mL. What dose will you administer to the patient?

   A. 3.5 mL
   B. 3 mL
   C. 4 mL
   D. 4.3 mL

CORRECT ANSWERS AND RATIONALES

1. A. 4 mL
2. C. 15 mL
3. B. 5 mL
4. A. True
5. C. 3 mL
6. C. 0.4 mL
7. D. 9 mL
8. A. 7.2 mL
9. D. 2.4 mL
10. A. 3.5 mL

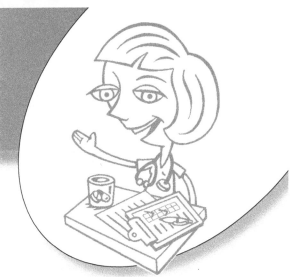

chapter **6**

Calculating Heparin Dose

Heparin is an anticoagulant (prevents the formation of blood clots) that is pre-scribed to patients who have venous thromboembolism, unstable angina, acute myocardial infarction, and other conditions that are associated with blood clots. Heparin is administered as a subcutaneous (S.C.) injection or administered intravenously and is also used to flush a Hep-Lock that connects intravenous (I.V.) tubing to the patient's vein.

So far nearly all dosages that you calculated throughout this book used met-ric units—milligrams, micrograms, and milliliters. Heparin is different and is measured in USP units (U), which is a standard set by the United States Pharmacopeial Convention Inc.

In this chapter you'll learn how to read a medication order for heparin and calculate the proper dose to administer to your patient.

1. A Close Look at Heparin

Heparin prevents blood from clotting, which is the goal if the patient is at risk for blood clots, but too much heparin can lead to excessive bleeding even from a slight injury. Therefore, it is important to maintain a **therapeutic level** of hepa-rin at all times.

The therapeutic level is a range that is measured using the **partial thrombo-plastin time** (PTT) test. A baseline PTT is taken before heparin is adminis-tered. The physician uses the test results to determine the dose to prescribe to the patient. Another PTT test is performed 4 hours to 12 hours after the hepa-rin is administered depending on the health care facility's policy. Based on the test results, the physician determines if any adjustments must be made to the dose.

If the patient has minor bleeding, then heparin is stopped and vital signs and complete blood count (CBC) is taken. However, if the patient experiences major bleeding, then the physician will likely to order **protamine** to reverse the effect of heparin. Protamine can cause an **anaphylactic reaction**.

NURSING ALERT

Heparin has a high potential for injuring the patient, so it is a good idea to have another registered nurse confirm your heparin calculation and double check your setting of the heparin I.V.

2. Calculating a Heparin Dose

Heparin-administered I.V. is ordered as units per hour(s). The pharmacy delivers heparin mixed with I.V. fluid such as normal saline or D5W. You must calculate the number of milliliters per hour to administer to your patient.

Here's an example of a heparin order:

Heparin 800 U per hour

The Heparin Dose Calculation Formula

The heparin calculation is a two-step process. First you must calculate number of heparin units in a milliliter of I.V. fluids. And then calculate the number of milliliters to administer per hour to the patient.

Here's the heparin formula.

1. Calculate the number of heparin units in a milliliter of I.V. fluids

$$\text{Heparin (U/mL)} = \frac{\text{on hand heparin (U)}}{\text{on hand (mL)}}$$

2. Calculate the number of milliliters to administer per hour

$$\text{Dose (mL/hr)} = \frac{\text{ordered heparin (U)}}{\text{heparin (U/hr)}}$$

Calculating Using the Heparin Dose Formula

Let's calculate the dose for heparin 800 U/hr. On hand is 25,000 U of heparin in 250 mL of D5W.

1. Insert the values in the first step of calculation.

$$\text{Heparin (U/mL)} = \frac{25000 \text{ (U)}}{250 \text{ (mL)}}$$

2. Calculate the number of heparin units in a milliliter.

$$\text{Heparin (U/mL)} = 100 \text{ U}$$

3. Insert values in the second step of calculation.

$$\text{Dose (mL/hr)} = \frac{800 \text{ U}}{100 \text{ U}}$$

4. Calculate the number of milliliters per hour to administer to the patient.

$$\text{Dose (mL/hr)} = 8 \text{ mL/hr}$$

3. Be Prepared for Different Types of Heparin Questions

Don't be surprised if you are given the infusion rate on an examination and then asked to calculate the number of units of heparin that the patient received. For example, you see this order on the examination written as:

25,000 U heparin in 250 cc of D5W infused at 7 mL/U

The formula used to calculate the units of heparin that the patient received is a variation of heparin calculation formula. Here it is:

$$\text{Heparin (U/mL)} = \frac{\text{ordered (U)}}{\text{ordered (mL)}}$$
$$\text{Heparin (U)} = \text{heparin (U/mL)} \times \text{ordered (mL/hr)}$$

Insert the values specified in the order into the formula and then calculate as shown here:

$$\text{Heparin (U/mL)} = \frac{25,000 \text{ U}}{250 \text{ mL}}$$
$$\text{Heparin (U)} = 100 \text{ U} \times 7 \text{ mL/hr}$$
$$\text{Heparin (U)} = 700 \text{ U}$$

Check your answer by using the heparin calculation formula. Assume that the physician ordered 700 U of heparin for the patient and that you have on hand 25,000 U of heparin in 250 mL of D5W. Insert these values into the heparin calculation formula and calculate the dose per hour. The dose per hour should be the same as dose per hour specified in the original order.

$$Heparin\ (U/mL) = \frac{25,000\ U}{250\ mL}$$

$$Dose\ (mL/hr) = \frac{700\ U}{100\ mL}$$

$$Dose\ (mL/hr) = 7\ mL/hr$$

4. The Heparin Subcutaneous Formula

Heparin can also be ordered as an S.C. injection. In the order, the physician specifies the number of units of heparin that the patient should receive. You must calculate the dose to administer to the patient using the heparin subcutaneous formula.

The heparin subcutaneous formula should look familiar to you because it is the same formula used to calculate doses for other medication that you learned in Chapter 2.

Here's the formula:

$$Dose = \frac{ordered}{on\ hand} \times quantity$$

Let's say the order reads:

Heparin 5000 U S.C. daily

The label reads heparin 20,000 U/mL. Here's how to calculate the dose:

1. Insert values into the formula.

$$Dose = \frac{5000\ U}{20,000} \times 1\ mL$$

2. Calculate.

$$Dose = 0.25\ U \times 1\ mL$$

$$Dose = 0.25\ mL$$

NURSING ALERT

Before administering heparin determine the number of units of heparin that the patient has received within the last 24 hours. If the total number of units including the next dose is greater than 40,000 units, then don't administer the next dose and notify the physician. Adult patients should not receive more than 40,000 units per 24-hour period.

CASE STUDY

CASE 1
Calculate the heparin dose for the following orders.

QUESTION 1. Medication order: heparin 600 U/hr
Medication label: 20,000 U heparin in 1000 mL normal saline
How many milliliters will be administered to the patient per hour?

QUESTION 2. Medication order: heparin 400 U/hr
Medication label: 20,000 U heparin in 2000 mL normal saline
How many milliliters will be administered to the patient per hour?

QUESTION 3. Medication order: heparin 200 U/hr
Medication label: 25,000 U heparin in 500 mL D5W
How many milliliters will be administered to the patient per hour?

QUESTION 4. Medication order: heparin 250 U/hr
Medication label: 25,000 U heparin in 1000 mL D5W
How many milliliters will be administered to the patient per hour?

QUESTION 5. Medication order: heparin 75 U/hr
Medication label: 25,000 U heparin in 2000 mL normal saline
How many milliliters will be administered to the patient per hour?

QUESTION 6. Medication order: heparin 300 U/hr
Medication label: 20,000 U heparin in 1000 mL D5W
How many milliliters will be administered to the patient per hour?

QUESTION 7. Medication order: heparin 800 U/hr
Medication label: 10,000 U heparin in 500 mL normal saline
How many milliliters will be administered to the patient per hour?

QUESTION 8. Medication order: heparin 400 U/hr
Medication label: 25,000 U heparin in 2000 mL D5W
How many milliliters will be administered to the patient per hour?

QUESTION 9. Medication order: heparin 700 U/hr
Medication label: 25,000 U heparin in 250 mL normal saline
How many milliliters will be administered to the patient per hour?

QUESTION 10. Medication order: heparin 300 U/hr
Medication label: 25,000 U heparin in 250 mL D5W
How many milliliters will be administered to the patient per hour?

ANSWERS

1. Heparin (U/mL) $= \dfrac{20,000\ U}{1000\ mL}$

    Dose (mL/hr) $= \dfrac{600\ U}{20\ U}$

    Dose (mL/hr) $= 30\ mL$

2. Heparin (U/mL) $= \dfrac{20,000\ U}{2000\ mL}$

    Dose (mL/hr) $= \dfrac{400\ U}{10\ U}$

    Dose (mL/hr) $= 40\ mL$

3. Heparin (U/mL) $= \dfrac{25,000\ U}{500\ mL}$

    Dose (mL/hr) $= \dfrac{200\ U}{50\ U}$

    Dose (mL/hr) $= 4\ mL$

4. Heparin (U/mL) $= \dfrac{25,000\ U}{1000\ mL}$

    Dose (mL/hr) $= \dfrac{250\ U}{25\ U}$

    Dose (mL/hr) $= 10\ mL$

5. Heparin (U/mL) $= \dfrac{25,000\ U}{2000\ mL}$

    Dose (mL/hr) $= \dfrac{75\ U}{12.5\ U}$

    Dose (mL/hr) $= 6\ mL$

6. Heparin (U/mL) $= \dfrac{20,000\ U}{1000\ mL}$

    Dose (mL/hr) $= \dfrac{300\ U}{20\ U}$

    Dose (mL/hr) $= 15\ mL$

7. $\text{Heparin (U/mL)} = \dfrac{10,000\ U}{500\ mL}$

$\text{Dose (mL/hr)} = \dfrac{800\ U}{20\ U}$

$\text{Dose (mL/hr)} = 40\ mL$

8. $\text{Heparin (U/mL)} = \dfrac{25,000\ U}{2000\ mL}$

$\text{Dose (mL/hr)} = \dfrac{400\ U}{12.5\ U}$

$\text{Dose (mL/hr)} = 32\ mL$

9. $\text{Heparin (U/mL)} = \dfrac{25,000\ U}{250\ mL}$

$\text{Dose (mL/hr)} = \dfrac{700\ U}{100\ U}$

$\text{Dose (mL/hr)} = 7\ mL$

10. $\text{Heparin (U/mL)} = \dfrac{25,000\ U}{250\ mL}$

$\text{Dose (mL/hr)} = \dfrac{300\ U}{100\ U}$

$\text{Dose (mL/hr)} = 3\ mL$

CASE STUDY

CASE 2
Calculate the correct doses using the heparin subcutaneous formula for the following orders.

QUESTION 1. Medication order: heparin 5000 U S.C. daily
Medication label: heparin 20,000 U/2 mL
How many milliliters will be administered to the patient?

QUESTION 2. Medication order: heparin 4000 U S.C. daily
Medication label: heparin 10,000 U/mL
How many milliliters will be administered to the patient?

QUESTION 3. Medication order: heparin 2500 U S.C. daily
Medication label: heparin 25,000 U/10 mL
How many milliliters will be administered to the patient?

QUESTION 4. Medication order: heparin 2000 U S.C. daily
Medication label: 20,000 U heparin/5 mL
How many milliliters will be administered to the patient?

QUESTION 5. Medication order: heparin 7500 U S.C. daily
Medication label: 20,000 U heparin/2 mL
How many milliliters will be administered to the patient?

QUESTION 6. Medication order: heparin 8000 U S.C. daily
Medication label: 20,000 U heparin/10 mL
How many milliliters will be administered to the patient?

QUESTION 7. Medication order: heparin 6250 U/hr
Medication label: 25,000 U heparin/4 mL
How many milliliters will be administered to the patient?

QUESTION 8. Medication order: heparin 4000 U S.C. daily
Medication label: 10,000 U heparin/5 mL
How many milliliters will be administered to the patient?

QUESTION 9. Medication order: heparin 3000 U S.C. daily
Medication label: 15,000 U heparin/5 mL
How many milliliters will be administered to the patient?

QUESTION 10. Medication order: heparin 6000 U S.C. daily
Medication label: 10,000 U heparin/5 mL
How many milliliters will be administered to the patient?

ANSWERS

1. $\text{Dose (mL/hr)} = \dfrac{5000 \text{ U}}{20,000 \text{ U}} \times 2 \text{ mL}$

   $\text{Dose (mL/hr)} = 0.25 \text{ U} \times 2 \text{ mL}$

   $\text{Dose (mL/hr)} = 0.5 \text{ mL}$

2. $\text{Dose (mL/hr)} = \dfrac{4000 \text{ U}}{10,000 \text{ U}} \times 1 \text{ mL}$

   $\text{Dose (mL/hr)} = 0.4 \text{ U} \times 1 \text{ mL}$

   $\text{Dose (mL/hr)} = 0.4 \text{ mL}$

3. Dose (mL/hr) $= \dfrac{2500\ U}{25{,}000\ U} \times 10\ mL$

   Dose (mL/hr) $= 0.1\ U \times 10\ mL$

   Dose (mL/hr) $= 1\ mL$

4. Dose (mL/hr) $= \dfrac{2000\ U}{20{,}000\ U} \times 5\ mL$

   Dose (mL/hr) $= 0.1\ U \times 5\ mL$

   Dose (mL/hr) $= 0.5\ mL$

5. Dose (mL/hr) $= \dfrac{7500\ U}{20{,}000\ U} \times 2\ mL$

   Dose (mL/hr) $= 0.375\ U \times 2\ mL$

   Dose (mL/hr) $= 0.75\ mL$

6. Dose (mL/hr) $= \dfrac{8000\ U}{20{,}000\ U} \times 10\ mL$

   Dose (mL/hr) $= 0.4\ U \times 10\ mL$

   Dose (mL/hr) $= 4\ mL$

7. Dose (mL/hr) $= \dfrac{6250\ U}{25{,}000\ U} \times 4\ mL$

   Dose (mL/hr) $= 0.25\ U \times 4\ mL$

   Dose (mL/hr) $= 1\ mL$

8. Dose (mL/hr) $= \dfrac{4000\ U}{10{,}000\ U} \times 5\ mL$

   Dose (mL/hr) $= 0.4\ U \times 5\ mL$

   Dose (mL/hr) $= 2\ mL$

9. Dose (mL/hr) $= \dfrac{3000\ U}{15{,}000\ U} \times 5\ mL$

   Dose (mL/hr) $= 0.2\ U \times 5\ mL$

   Dose (mL/hr) $= 1\ mL$

10. Dose (mL/hr) $= \dfrac{6000\ U}{10{,}000\ U} \times 5\ mL$

    Dose (mL/hr) $= 0.6\ U \times 5\ mL$

    Dose (mL/hr) $= 3\ mL$

FINAL CHECK-UP

1. The physician ordered heparin 500 U/hr. The medication label reads 20,000 U heparin in 200-mL normal saline. How many milliliters will be administered to the patient per hour?

   A. 50 mL

   B. 500 mL

   C. 5 mL

   D. 0.5 mL

2. The physician ordered heparin 800 U/hr. The medication label reads 25,000 U heparin in 250-mL D5W. How many milliliters will be administered to the patient per hour?

   A. 7.5 mL

   B. 7 mL

   C. 8 mL

   D. 8.5 mL

3. The physician ordered heparin 6000 U S.C. The medication label reads 10,000 U heparin/10 mL. How many milliliters will be administered to the patient?

   A. 5 mL

   B. 6 mL

   C. 6.5 mL

   D. 7 mL

4. The physician ordered heparin 20,000 U/hr. The medication label reads 2000 U heparin in 20-mL normal saline. Two milliliters will be administered to the patient per hour.

   A. True

   B. False

5. The physician ordered heparin 5250 U S.C. The medication label reads 15,000 U heparin/5 mL. How many milliliters will be administered to the patient per hour?

   A. 1.25 mL

   B. 1 mL

   C. 1.75 mL

   D. 2 mL

6. The physician ordered heparin 400 U/hr. The medication label reads 20,000 U heparin in 400-mL normal saline. How many milliliters will be administered to the patient per hour?

   A. 9 mL

   B. 8 mL

   C. 7 mL

   D. 6 mL

7. The physician ordered heparin 100 U/hr. The medication label reads 20,000 U heparin in 2000 mL D5W. How many milliliters will be administered to the patient per hour?

   A. 1 mL

   B. 1.9 mL

   C. 0.9 mL

   D. 10 mL

8. The physician ordered heparin 4500 U S.C. The medication label reads 10,000 U heparin-5 mL. How many milliliters will be administered to the patient per hour?

   A. 2.25 mL

   B. 2.50 mL

   C. 2 mL

   D. 3 mL

9. The physician ordered heparin 600 U/hr. The medication label reads 25,000 U heparin in 500-mL normal saline. How many milliliters will be administered to the patient per hour?

   A. 0.2 mL

   B. 1.2 mL

   C. 0.12 mL

   D. 12 mL

10. The physician ordered heparin 800 U/hr. The medication label reads 10,000 U heparin in 250-mL D5W. How many milliliters will be administered to the patient per hour?

   A. 20 mL

   B. 2.1 mL

   C. 2 mL

   D. 21 mL

CORRECT ANSWERS AND RATIONALES

1. C. 5 mL
2. C. 8 mL
3. B. 6 mL
4. A. True
5. C. 1.75 mL
6. B. 8 mL
7. D. 10 mL
8. A. 2.25 mL
9. D. 12 mL
10. A. 20 mL

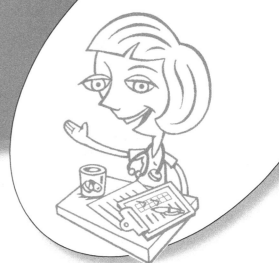

Calculating Dopamine Dose

LEARNING OBJECTIVES

> **KEY TERM**
>
> Calculating Using the Dopamine Dose
>   Calculation Formula

Dopamine is a neurotransmitter formed in the brain that affects movement, emotion, and perception. An imbalance or absence of dopamine can result in the patient having unnatural movement, irrational thoughts, and other signs and symptoms associated with Parkinson disease, bipolar disorder, schizophrenia, and paranoia. Physicians prescribe dopamine to bring dopamine into balance and return the patient to normal movement, emotions, and perceptions. Dopamine is also frequently prescribed for kidney perfusion and for coronary conditions.

Calculating the proper dose of dopamine to administer to your patient is a little different from the way you calculate the dose of other medications because the prescribed dose is per kilogram and the medication on hand is a concentration. A concentration is a mixture of intravenous (I.V.) fluid that contains a specific amount of dopamine.

Before you calculate the dose for your patient, you must use the prescribed dose to calculate prescribed dose for your patient's weight and you also need to calculate the amount of dopamine in a milliliter of the concentration. You'll learn these calculations in this chapter.

1. Calculating Dopamine Dose

There are several steps that you must perform to calculate the proper dose of **dopamine** to administer to your patient. Nearly all you used to calculate other medication throughout this book.

Dopamine is prescribed by weight similar to pediatric medication (see Chapter 5). The physician prescribes a dose per kilogram of the patient's weight, which means that you'll have to convert the patient's weight from pounds to kilograms in order to calculate the dose to administer to the patient.

Dopamine is administered intravenously using an infusion pump. The dose prescribed by the physician is for a minute infusion. The dose entered into I.V. infusion pumps is for an hour of infusion, which requires you to adjust the prescribed dose from a minute to an hour.

Dopamine comes premixed in an I.V. fluid from the pharmacy. You must calculate the **concentration** of dopamine in a milliliter of I.V. fluid, which is then used to calculate the dose of dopamine to administer to the patient.

Here's an example of a dopamine order:

$$\text{Dopamine 3 mcg/kg} \cdot \text{min}$$

2. The Dopamine Dose Calculation Formula

There are three steps in calculating the dose of dopamine to administer to your patient. The first step is to convert your patient's weight to kilograms, if your patient's weight is recorded in pounds. You'll recall from Chapter 5 that 1 kg = 2.2 lb. Convert your patient's weight from pounds to kilograms by dividing your patient's weight in pounds by 2.2.

The second step is to calculate the concentration of dopamine in 1 mL of I.V. fluid. This is similar to calculating the concentration of heparin that you learned to do in Chapter 6. The I.V. solution container specifies the total amount of milliliters and the total amount of dopamine in the container. You need to calculate the concentration of dopamine in 1 mL of I.V. fluid. You do this by dividing the amount of dopamine in the I.V. container by the amount of I.V. fluid. The result is the concentration—the number of milligrams of dopamine in 1 mL of I.V. fluid.

The third step is to calculate the dose to administer to your patient.

Here's the dopamine formula:

1. Convert the patient's weight from pounds to kilograms.

$$\text{Weight (kg)} = \frac{\text{weight (lb)}}{2.2}$$

2. Calculate the concentration of dopamine that is delivered from the pharmacy.

$$\text{Concentration} = \frac{\text{on hand (mg)}}{\text{on hand (mL)}}$$

3. Calculate the dose to administer to your patient. Remember that the prescribed dose is for 1 minute and that the infusion pump is set for 1 hour. Therefore, you must multiply by 60 minutes.

$$\text{Dose (mL/hr)} = \frac{\text{ordered (mg)} \times \text{weight (kg)} \times 60 \text{ minute}}{\text{concentration}}$$

> **NURSING ALERT**
>
> The prescribed dose of dopamine might be in micrograms (mcg) and the I.V. solution delivered by the pharmacy has dopamine in milligrams (mg). Therefore, you must convert the amount of dopamine in the I.V. bag from milligrams to micrograms before calculating the dose to administer to your patients. You convert milligrams to micrograms by multiplying the milligrams by 1000 (see Chapter 2 Converting Metric Units).

Calculating Using the Dopamine Dose Calculation Formula

Say that the practitioner wrote the following prescription for your patient who weighs 165 lb:

$$\text{Dopamine 3 mcg/kg} \cdot \text{min}$$

The pharmacy delivered an I.V. labeled dopamine 400 mg in 250 D5W. Here's how to calculate the dose to administer to your patient:

1. Convert your patient's weight from pounds to kilograms.

$$75 \text{ kg} = \frac{165 \text{ lb}}{2.2 \text{ lb}}$$

2. Calculate the dopamine concentration in the I.V. fluid.

$$400,000 \text{ mcg} = 400 \text{ mg} \times 1000$$
$$1600 \text{ mcg} = \frac{400,000}{250 \text{ mL}}$$

3. Calculate the dose.

$$\text{Dose (mL/hr)} = \frac{3 \text{ mcg} \times 75 \text{ kg} \times 60 \text{ minute}}{1600 \text{ mcg}}$$

$$\text{Dose (mL/hr)} = \frac{225 \text{ mcg} \times 60 \text{ minute}}{1600 \text{ mcg}}$$

$$\text{Dose (mL/hr)} = \frac{13,500 \text{ mcg}}{1600 \text{ mcg}}$$

$$\text{Dose (mL/hr)} = 8.437 = 8 \text{ mL/hr}$$

CASE STUDY

CASE 1

Calculate the correct dose for the following dopamine orders.

QUESTION 1. Medication order: dopamine 5 mcg/kg · min for a patient that weighs 178 lb
Medication label: dopamine 800 mg in 500 D5W
How many milliliters will be administered to the patient per hour?

QUESTION 2. Medication order: dopamine 7 mcg/kg · min for a patient that weighs 190 lb
Medication label: dopamine 800 mg in 500 D5W
How many milliliters will be administered to the patient per hour?

QUESTION 3. Medication order: dopamine 8 mcg/kg · min for a patient that weighs 165 lb
Medication label: dopamine 400 mg in 250 D5W
How many milliliters will be administered to the patient per hour?

QUESTION 4. Medication order: dopamine 4 mcg/kg · min for a patient that weighs 184 lb
Medication label: dopamine 400 mg in 250 D5W
How many milliliters will be administered to the patient per hour?

QUESTION 5. Medication order: dopamine 7 mcg/kg · min for a patient that weighs 155 lb
Medication label: dopamine 800 mg in 500 D5W
How many milliliters will be administered to the patient per hour?

QUESTION 6. Medication order: dopamine 5 mcg/kg · min for a patient that weighs 175 lb
Medication label: dopamine 400 mg in 250 D5W
How many milliliters will be administered to the patient per hour?

QUESTION 7. Medication order: dopamine 7 mcg/kg · min for a patient that weighs 190 lb
Medication label: dopamine 800 mg in 500 D5W
How many milliliters will be administered to the patient per hour?

QUESTION 8. Medication order: dopamine 5 mcg/kg · min for a patient that weighs 185 lb
Medication label: dopamine 400 mg in 250 D5W
How many milliliters will be administered to the patient per hour?

QUESTION 9. Medication order: dopamine 3 mcg/kg · min for a patient that weighs 172 lb

Medication label: dopamine 400 mg in 250 D5W

How many milliliters will be administered to the patient per hour?

QUESTION 10. Medication order: dopamine 5 mcg/kg · min for a patient that weighs 200 lb

Medication label: dopamine 800 mg in 500 D5W

How many milliliters will be administered to the patient per hour?

ANSWERS

1. $80.909 \text{ kg} = \dfrac{178 \text{ lb}}{2.2 \text{ lb}}$

$800{,}000 \text{ mcg} = 800 \text{ mg} \times 1000$

$1600 \text{ mcg} = \dfrac{800{,}000 \text{ mcg}}{500 \text{ mL}}$

$\text{Dose (mL/hr)} = \dfrac{5 \text{ mcg} \times 80.909 \text{ kg} \times 60 \text{ minutes}}{1600 \text{ mcg}}$

$\text{Dose (mL/hr)} = \dfrac{404.545 \text{ mcg} \times 60 \text{ minutes}}{1600 \text{ mcg}}$

$\text{Dose (mL/hr)} = \dfrac{24{,}272.7 \text{ mcg}}{1600 \text{ mcg}}$

$\text{Dose (mL/hr)} = 15.17 = 15 \text{ mL/hr}$

2. $86.363 \text{ kg} = \dfrac{190 \text{ lb}}{2.2 \text{ lb}}$

$800{,}000 \text{ mcg} = 800 \text{ mg} \times 1000$

$1600 \text{ mcg} = \dfrac{800{,}000 \text{ mcg}}{500 \text{ mL}}$

$\text{Dose (mL/hr)} = \dfrac{7 \text{ mcg} \times 86.363 \text{ kg} \times 60 \text{ minutes}}{1600 \text{ mcg}}$

$\text{Dose (mL/hr)} = \dfrac{604.54 \text{ mcg} \times 60 \text{ minutes}}{1600 \text{ mcg}}$

$\text{Dose (mL/hr)} = \dfrac{36{,}272.5}{1600 \text{ mcg}}$

$\text{Dose (mL/hr)} = 22.67 = 23 \text{ mL/hr}$

3. $$75 \text{ kg} = \frac{165 \text{ lb}}{2.2 \text{ lb}}$$

$$400{,}000 \text{ mcg} = 400 \text{ mg} \times 1000$$

$$1600 \text{ mcg} = \frac{400{,}000 \text{ mcg}}{250 \text{ mL}}$$

$$\text{Dose (mL/hr)} = \frac{8 \text{ mcg} \times 75 \text{ kg} \times 60 \text{ minutes}}{1600 \text{ mcg}}$$

$$\text{Dose (mL/hr)} = \frac{600 \text{ mcg} \times 60 \text{ minutes}}{1600 \text{ mcg}}$$

$$\text{Dose (mL/hr)} = \frac{36{,}000 \text{ mcg}}{1600 \text{ mcg}}$$

$$\text{Dose (mL/hr)} = 22.5 = 23 \text{ mL/hr}$$

4. $$83.636 \text{ kg} = \frac{184 \text{ lb}}{2.2 \text{ lb}}$$

$$400{,}000 \text{ mcg} = 400 \text{ mg} \times 1000$$

$$1600 \text{ mcg} = \frac{400{,}000 \text{ mcg}}{250 \text{ mL}}$$

$$\text{Dose (mL/hr)} = \frac{4 \text{ mcg} \times 83.636 \text{ kg} \times 60 \text{ minutes}}{1600 \text{ mcg}}$$

$$\text{Dose (mL/hr)} = \frac{334.544 \text{ mcg} \times 60 \text{ minutes}}{1600 \text{ mcg}}$$

$$\text{Dose (mL/hr)} = \frac{20{,}072.64 \text{ mcg}}{1600 \text{ mcg}}$$

$$\text{Dose (mL/hr)} = 12.545 = 13 \text{ mL/hr}$$

5. $$70.454 \text{ kg} = \frac{155 \text{ lb}}{2.2 \text{ lb}}$$

$$800{,}000 \text{ mcg} = 800 \text{ mg} \times 1000$$

$$1600 \text{ mcg} = \frac{800{,}000 \text{ mcg}}{500 \text{ mL}}$$

$$\text{Dose (mL/hr)} = \frac{7 \text{ mcg} \times 70.454 \text{ kg} \times 60 \text{ minutes}}{1600 \text{ mcg}}$$

$$\text{Dose (mL/hr)} = \frac{493.178 \text{ mcg} \times 60 \text{ minutes}}{1600 \text{ mcg}}$$

$$\text{Dose (mL/hr)} = \frac{29{,}590.68 \text{ mcg}}{1600 \text{ mcg}}$$

$$\text{Dose (mL/hr)} = 18.494 = 19 \text{ mL/hr}$$

6. $79.545 \text{ kg} = \dfrac{175 \text{ lb}}{2.2 \text{ lb}}$

$400,000 \text{ mcg} = 400 \text{ mg} \times 1000$

$1600 \text{ mcg} = \dfrac{400,000 \text{ mcg}}{250 \text{ mL}}$

$\text{Dose (mL/hr)} = \dfrac{5 \text{ mcg} \times 79.545 \text{ kg} \times 60 \text{ minutes}}{1600 \text{ mcg}}$

$\text{Dose (mL/hr)} = \dfrac{397.725 \text{ mcg} \times 60 \text{ minutes}}{1600 \text{ mcg}}$

$\text{Dose (mL/hr)} = \dfrac{23,863.5 \text{ mcg}}{1600 \text{ mcg}}$

$\text{Dose (mL/hr)} = 14.914 = 15 \text{ mL/hr}$

7. $86.363 \text{ kg} = \dfrac{190 \text{ lb}}{2.2 \text{ lb}}$

$800,000 \text{ mcg} = 800 \text{ mg} \times 1000$

$1600 \text{ mcg} = \dfrac{800,000 \text{ mcg}}{500 \text{ mL}}$

$\text{Dose (mL/hr)} = \dfrac{7 \text{ mcg} \times 86.363 \text{ kg} \times 60 \text{ minutes}}{1600 \text{ mcg}}$

$\text{Dose (mL/hr)} = \dfrac{604.541 \text{ mcg} \times 60 \text{ minutes}}{1600 \text{ mcg}}$

$\text{Dose (mL/hr)} = \dfrac{36,272.46 \text{ mcg}}{1600 \text{ mcg}}$

$\text{Dose (mL/hr)} = 22.67 = 23 \text{ mL/hr}$

8. $84.09 \text{ kg} = \dfrac{185 \text{ lb}}{2.2 \text{ lb}}$

$400,000 \text{ mcg} = 400 \text{ mg} \times 1000$

$1600 \text{ mcg} = \dfrac{400,000 \text{ mcg}}{250 \text{ mL}}$

$\text{Dose (mL/hr)} = \dfrac{5 \text{ mcg} \times 84.09 \text{ kg} \times 60 \text{ minutes}}{1600 \text{ mcg}}$

$\text{Dose (mL/hr)} = \dfrac{420.45 \text{ mcg} \times 60 \text{ minutes}}{1600 \text{ mcg}}$

$\text{Dose (mL/hr)} = \dfrac{25,227 \text{ mcg}}{1600 \text{ mcg}}$

$\text{Dose (mL/hr)} = 15.766 = 16 \text{ mL/hr}$

9. $78.181\,kg = \dfrac{172\,lb}{2.2\,lb}$

$400{,}000\,mcg = 400\,mg \times 1000$

$1600\,mcg = \dfrac{400{,}000\,mcg}{250\,mL}$

$Dose\,(mL/hr) = \dfrac{3\,mcg \times 78.181\,kg \times 60\,minutes}{1600\,mcg}$

$Dose\,(mL/hr) = \dfrac{234.543\,mcg \times 60\,minutes}{1600\,mcg}$

$Dose\,(mL/hr) = \dfrac{14{,}072.58\,mcg}{1600\,mcg}$

$Dose\,(mL/hr) = 8.795 = 9\,mL/hr$

10. $90.909\,kg = \dfrac{200\,lb}{2.2\,lb}$

$800{,}000\,mcg = 800\,mg \times 1000$

$1600\,mcg = \dfrac{800{,}000\,mcg}{500\,mL}$

$Dose\,(mL/hr) = \dfrac{5\,mcg \times 90.909\,kg \times 60\,minutes}{1600\,mcg}$

$Dose\,(mL/hr) = \dfrac{454.545\,mcg \times 60\,minutes}{1600\,mcg}$

$Dose\,(mL/hr) = \dfrac{27{,}272.7\,mcg}{1600\,mcg}$

$Dose\,(mL/hr) = 17.045 = 17\,mL/hr$

FINAL CHECK-UP

1. The physician ordered dopamine 8 mcg/kg · min for a patient that weighs 220 lb. The pharmacy delivers dopamine 400 mg in 250 D5W. How many milliliters per hour will you set the infusion pump?

A. 30 mL

B. 29.5 mL

C. 31 mL

D. 29 mL

2. The physician ordered dopamine 3 mcg/kg · min for a patient that weighs 132 lb. The pharmacy delivers dopamine 400 mg in 250 D5W. How many milliliters per hour will you set the infusion pump?

   A. 6.5 mL

   B. 6.25 mL

   C. 6 mL

   D. 6.75 mL

3. The physician ordered dopamine 6 mcg/kg · min for a patient that weighs 154 lb. The pharmacy delivers dopamine 800 mg in 500 D5W. How many milliliters per hour will you set the infusion pump?

   A. 15 mL

   B. 16 mL

   C. 14 mL

   D. 17 mL

4. The physician ordered dopamine 5 mcg/kg · min for a patient that weighs 187 lb. The pharmacy delivers dopamine 400 mg in 250 D5W. The infusion pump should be set to 16 mL per hour.

   A. True

   B. False

5. The physician ordered dopamine 3 mcg/kg · min for a patient that weighs 131 lb. The pharmacy delivers dopamine 800 mg in 500 D5W. How many milliliters per hour will you set the infusion pump?

   A. 7 mL

   B. 6 mL

   C. 6.7 mL

   D. 6.8 mL

6. The physician ordered dopamine 7 mcg/kg · min for a patient that weighs 240 lb. The pharmacy delivers dopamine 400 mg in 250 D5W. How many milliliters per hour will you set the infusion pump?

   A. 28 mL

   B. 29 mL

   C. 28.6 mL

   D. 28.63 mL

7. The physician ordered dopamine 3 mcg/kg · min for a patient that weighs 180 lb. The pharmacy delivers dopamine 400 mg in 250 D5W. How many milliliters per hour will you set the infusion pump?

   A. 10 mL

   B. 9.2 mL

C. 9 mL

D. 9.5 mL

8. The physician ordered dopamine 4 mcg/kg · min for a patient that weighs
195 lb. The pharmacy delivers dopamine 800 mg in 500 D5W. How many
milliliters per hour will you set the infusion pump?

A. 13 mL

B. 14 mL

C. 13.7 mL

D. 13.29 mL

9. The physician ordered dopamine 5 mcg/kg · min for a patient that weighs
171 lb. The pharmacy delivers dopamine 800 mg in 500 D5W. How many
milliliters per hour will you set the infusion pump?

A. 1.5 mL

B. 14.6 mL

C. 14 mL

D. 15 mL

10. The physician ordered dopamine 5 mcg/kg · min for a patient that weighs
215 lb. The pharmacy delivers dopamine 400 mg in 250 D5W. How many
milliliters per hour will you set the infusion pump?

A. 18.715 mL

B. 18.71 mL

C. 18.3 mL

D. 18 mL

CORRECT ANSWERS AND RATIONALES

1. A. 30 mL

2. D. 6.75 mL

3. B. 16 mL

4. A. True

5. A. 7 mL

6. B. 29 mL

7. B. 9.2 mL

8. A. 13 mL

9. B. 14.6 mL

10. A. 18.3 mL

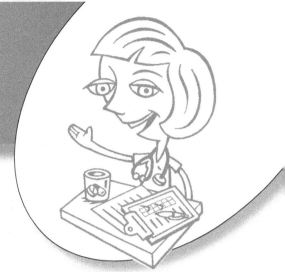

chapter **8**

Calculating Dose for Children Using Body Surface Area

Weight-based dose calculations, which you learned in Chapter 5, references one measurement of a child—weight—to calculate the proper dose. Some physicians prefer to use the child's body surface area (BSA) rather than weight as the basis for calculating the dose.

Body surface area reflects both the child's weight and height and is considered to be the most accurate way to calculate a dose for a child because it considers two measurement of a child.

In this chapter you'll learn how to calculate the proper dose of medication for your young patient by using the child's BSA.

1. What Is Body Surface Area?

Remember back in grammar school math when the teacher asked how many 1-ft square tiles are needed to cover the area of the kitchen floor. The teacher was really asking you to calculate the **surface area** of the kitchen floor.

Think of the surface area of a person as being similar to the surface area of the kitchen floor—with some obvious exceptions. The person's body has a relatively irregular shape and has more than two dimensions. You can't simply take a rule and measure every foot of the body like you can for the kitchen floor.

However, aside from these differences, there are similarities between the surface area of the kitchen floor and the surface area of a person's body. Both have an area that covers it (i.e., the floor and the body) called the surface area. And the surface area can be calculated using a mathematical formula, although a different formula is used to calculate the surface area of the body than is used to calculate the surface area of the kitchen floor.

Why Calculate the Surface Area?

After a medication is administered and absorbed into the body, the body breaks down the medication into components, which is referred to as metabolizing the medication. The components enter the bloodstream where they are distributed throughout the body and eventually excreted.

The rate at which the medication is metabolized influences the dose that is prescribed to the patient. The goal is for the physician to prescribe a dose that achieves a therapeutic level without resulting in an overdose.

If the dose is too high for **metabolism**, then this could lead to an overdose because a second dose is administered before the first dose is fully metabolized. If the dose is too low for the metabolism, then the medication could be excreted before the next dose is administered resulting in the medication never reaching a therapeutic level in the blood.

The patient's **metabolic mass** influences the rate at which the medication is metabolized. While the patient's weight is a good indicator of a patient's metabolic mass, the patient's **body surface area** is even a better indicator of metabolic mass.

Therefore, some physicians prefer to use body surface area rather than weight to prescribe medication. This is especially true when highly sensitive medication such as chemotherapy is being prescribed.

2. Calculating the Body Surface Area

Unfortunately, the formula for calculating the body surface area is more complicated than the formula used to calculate how many 1-ft tiles are needed to cover the kitchen floor. There are several formulas that can be used to calculate the **BSA**. The **Du Bois & Du Bois formula** is commonly used. Here it is:

$$BSA = (71.84 \times \text{weight (kg)}^{0.425} \times \text{height (cm)}^{0.725})/10{,}000$$

But don't sweat the math because the math to calculate the body surface area is done for you if you use **West nomogram** (Figure 8–1). A nomogram is a chart that shows the relationship among values. The West nomogram shows the relationship among the patient's height, weight, and body surface area.

The West nomogram is divided into three sets of numbers. The first set is height in inches, the second set is body surface, and the third set is weight in pounds. These sets are lined up together based on the Du Bois & Du Bois formula.

Here's how to use the West nomogram to calculate the patient's body surface area:

1. Measure the patient's height in centimeters or inches.

2. Weight the patient in kilogram or pounds.

3. Draw a line from the patient's height in the height set of numbers on the West nomogram to the patient's weight in the weight set of numbers.

4. The line intersects a number on the body surface set of numbers. This is the patient's body surface area in **square meters** (m^2).

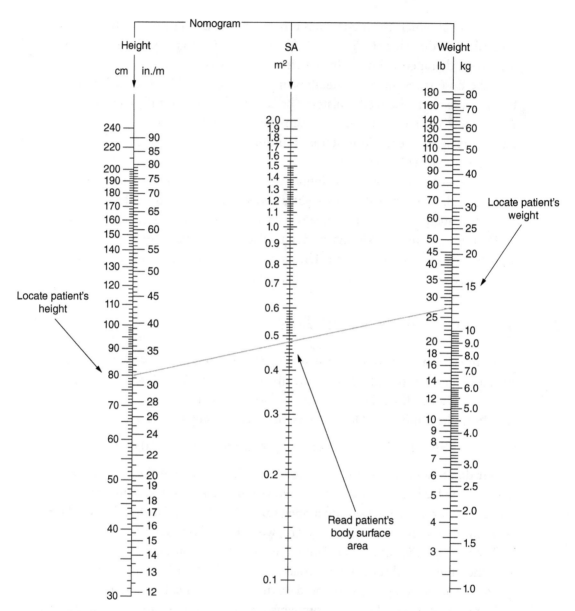

FIGURE 8–1 · Draw a line from the patient's height to the patient's weight on the West nomogram and the line intersects the patient's body surface. *(Modified from data of E. Boyd by C.D. West; from Behrman, R.E., Kliegman, R.M., & Jenson, H.B. (eds.): Nelson Textbook of Pediatrics, 16th ed. Philadelphia, PA, W.B. Saunders, 2000.)*

3. The BSA Child Dose Calculation Formula

You probably realize that an **adult dose** of a medication is too much of a dose to administer to a child because the child is much smaller than the adult. Then what is the proper dose for a child?

You determine the proper dose for a child by using the following formula that uses both the child's body surface area and the adult dose:

$$\text{Child dose} = \frac{\text{body surface area } (m^2)}{1.73 \ m^2} \times \text{adult dose}$$

Calculating Using the Formula

Let's say that the child is 32 in tall and weighs 25 lb. The physician orders Demerol with the adult dose of 100 mg. Your job is to calculate the dose to administer to the child.

1. Determine the child's body surface area. You do this by drawing a line from 32 in in the height set of number to 25 lb in the weight set of numbers on the West nomogram. In doing so, you'll notice that the line intersects 0.50 m^2 in the body surface set of numbers. This is the child's body surface area.

2. Enter the body surface area and the adult dose into the formula.

$$\text{Child dose} = \frac{0.5 \ m^2}{1.73 \ m^2} \times 100 \ \text{mg}$$

3. Divide the child's body surface area by 1.73 m^2.

$$\text{Child dose} = 0.289 \times 100 \ \text{mg}$$

4. Multiply the adult dose by 0.289 to arrive at the child's dose.

$$\text{Child dose} = 28.9 \ \text{mg}$$

NURSING ALERT

Think of 0.289 or whatever value is calculated as the percentage of the adult dose. In this example, the child's dose based on this child's body surface area is 28.9% of the adult dose. Remember that this percentage changes based on the child's body surface.

CASE STUDY

CASE 1
Calculate the correct doses using the BSA child dose calculation formula for the following orders.

QUESTION 1. The child is 85 cm tall and weighs 25 lb and the adult dose of Capoten is 6.25 mg.
How many milligrams will be administered to your patient?

QUESTION 2. The child is 42 in tall and weighs 40 lb and the adult dose of Decadron is 3 mg.
How many milligrams will be administered to your patient?

QUESTION 3. The child is 44 in tall and weighs 50 lb and the adult dose of Cephalexin is 125 mg.
How many milligrams will be administered to your patient?

QUESTION 4. The child is 70 cm tall and weighs 9 kg and the adult dose of Zovirax is 25 mg.
How many milligrams will be administered to your patient?

QUESTION 5. The child is 45 cm in tall and weighs 3 kg and the adult dose of Celocin is 125 mg.
How many milligrams will be administered to your patient?

QUESTION 6. The child is 21 in tall and weighs 10 lb and the adult dose of Zofran is 2000 mcg.
How many milligrams will be administered to your patient?

QUESTION 7. The child is 75 in tall and weighs 25 lb and the adult dose of Ampicillin is 100 mg.
How many milligrams will be administered to your patient?

QUESTION 8. The child is 41 in tall and weighs 60 lb and the adult dose of Lithostat is 250 mg.
How many milligrams will be administered to your patient?

QUESTION 9. The child is 105 cm tall and weighs 25 kg and the adult dose of Benylin is 50 mg.
How many milligrams will be administered to your patient?

QUESTION 10. The child is 80 cm tall and weighs 25 lb and the adult dose of Amoxicillin is 125 mg.
How many milligrams will be administered to your patient?

ANSWERS

1. $1.8\,mg = \dfrac{0.5\,m^2}{1.73\,m^2} \times 6.25\,mg$

2. $1.3\,mg = \dfrac{0.75\,m^2}{1.73\,m^2} \times 3\,mg$

3. $61.4\,mg = \dfrac{0.85\,m^2}{1.73\,m^2} \times 125\,mg$

4. $5.8\,mg = \dfrac{0.4\,m^2}{1.73\,m^2} \times 25\,mg$

5. $13\,mg = \dfrac{0.18\,m^2}{1.73\,m^2} \times 125\,mg$

6. $289\,mcg = \dfrac{0.25\,m^2}{1.73\,m^2} \times 2000\,mcg$

7. $27.2\,mg = \dfrac{0.47\,m^2}{1.73\,m^2} \times 100\,mg$

8. $122.8\,mg = \dfrac{0.85\,m^2}{1.73\,m^2} \times 250\,mg$

9. $24\,mg = \dfrac{0.83\,m^2}{1.73\,m^2} \times 50\,mg$

10. $35.4\,mg = \dfrac{0.49\,m^2}{1.73\,m^2} \times 125\,mg$

FINAL CHECK-UP

1. **The adult dose ordered is Tegopen 125 mg for a patient who is 70 cm tall and weighs 20 lb. What dose would you administer to the patient?**
   A. 32.5 mg
   B. 33.5 mg
   C. 30.1 mg
   D. 31.2 mg

2. The adult dose ordered is Ampicillin 100 mg for a patient who is 45 cm tall and weighs 7 lb. What dose would you administer to the patient?
   A. 10 mg
   B. 12.5 mg
   C. 11.6 mg
   D. 11 mg

3. The adult dose ordered is Cefotan 50 mg for a patient who is 30 in tall and weighs 25 lb. What dose would you administer to the patient?
   A. 13.8 mg
   B. 14.5 mg
   C. 13.7 mg
   D. 14 mg

4. The adult dose ordered is Ketzol 25 mg for a patient who is 36 in tall and weighs 15 kg. What dose would you administer to the patient?
   A. 8.7 mg
   B. 8 mg
   C. 8.5 mg
   D. 7.8 mg

5. The adult dose ordered is Erythrocin 50 mg for a patient who is 48 in tall and weighs 70 lb. What dose would you administer to the patient?
   A. 31.8 mg
   B. 28 mg
   C. 30 mg
   D. 29.8 mg

6. The adult dose ordered is Tetracycline 250 mg for a patient who is 43 in tall and weighs 25 kg. What dose would you administer to the patient?
   A. 96.1 mg
   B. 86.7 mg
   C. 84.1 mg
   D. 90.2 mg

7. The adult dose ordered is Trovan 100 mg for a patient who is 38 in tall and weighs 45 lb. What dose would you administer to the patient?
   A. 42 mg
   B. 42.1 mg
   C. 46.2 mg
   D. 42.3 mg

8. The adult dose ordered is Bactrim 30 mg for a patient who is 86 cm tall and weighs 30 lb. What dose would you administer to the patient?

   A. 10.4 mg

   B. 9.6 mg

   C. 9 mg

   D. 11.1 mg

9. The adult dose ordered is Sporanox 200 mg for a patient who is 60 cm tall and weighs 7 kg. What dose would you administer to the patient?

   A. 36 mg

   B. 37.1 mg

   C. 36.9 mg

   D. 40.5 mg

10. The adult dose ordered is Flagyl 500 mg for a patient who is 70 cm tall and weighs 9 kg. What dose would you administer to the patient?

    A. 131.1 mg

    B. 128.7 mg

    C. 127.1 mg

    D. 130 mg

CORRECT ANSWERS AND RATIONALES

1. A. 32.5 mg

2. C. 11.6 mg

3. B. 14.5 mg

4. A. 8.7 mg

5. A. 31.8 mg

6. B. 86.7 mg

7. C. 46.2 mg

8. A. 10.4 mg

9. D. 40.5 mg

10. D. 130 mg

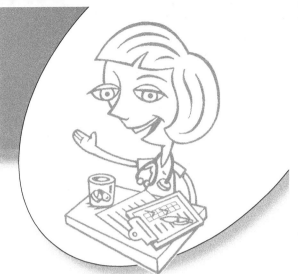

chapter 9

Enteral Tube Feeding

KEY TERMS

Calculating Using the Enteral Tube   Enteral Tube Feeding Concentration
  Feeding Formula
Calculating Using the Enteral Tube
  Feeding Formula by Caloric Intake

Patients who have a cardiovascular accident (CVA), tracheoesophageal fistula, esophageal atresia, or other conditions that affect swallowing are at risk for aspiration pneumonia and malnutrition. Physicians take the preemptive strategy of placing the patient on enteral tube feeding, which greatly reduces the risk for aspiration and assures that nutrients reach the stomach.

Enteral tube feedings usually come in full strength; however, the physician typically orders enteral tube feedings at less than full strength. This requires you to dilute the enteral tube feeding before it is administered to your patient.

In this chapter you'll learn how to calculate the fraction or percentage of dilution that must be applied to the full concentration of the enteral tube feeding.

1. What Is Enteral Tube Feeding?

There are a number of conditions that can temporarily or permanently interfere with a patient's ability to swallow, placing the patient at risk for **malnutrition** and depletion of fat and muscle. In order to reduce this risk, the patient's physician orders the insertion of a feeding tube and **enteral tube** feeding.

There are following two types of feeding tubes:

- Nasogastric feeding tube: The **nasogastric feeding tube** is commonly called an **NG tube** and is used for short-term enteral tube feedings. The NG tube passes through the patient's nares, then the esophagus, and into the stomach. Nutrients flow through the NG tube and go directly into the stomach without touching or affecting the esophagus.

- Gastric feeding tube: The **gastric feeding tube** is commonly called the **percutaneous endoscopic gastrostomy (PEG)** tube. The PEG tube is surgically placed through the abdominal wall and into the stomach. The PEG tube is held in place by either a balloon tip or by a retention dome. PEG tubes are replaced about every 6 months.

Enteral Tube Feeding Concentration

Imagine having a bottle of 100% orange juice. You can drink an 8-oz glass without having any uncomfortable feeling because you can tolerate 100% orange juice. However, someone else may not tolerate it as well, but does not have adverse effects if the 8-oz glass has 50% orange juice and 50% water. The problem is that the bottle contains 100% orange juice. This means that the orange juice must be diluted before being ingested.

This is similar in concept with enteral tube feedings except the feedings aren't orange juice. Depending on the patient's needs, the physician may order a special blend of nutrients that is prepared by the pharmacy, which meets the patient's requirements. Other times, the physician may order enteral tube feedings that are prepackaged, which may need to be diluted before being administered to the patient. You must calculate the dilution and prepare the enteral tube feeding.

2. Enteral Tube Feeding Formula

The physician will prescribe the strength of the prepackaged enteral food feeding that is to be administered to the patient. Prepackaged enteral food feeding is 100% and the strength ordered by the physician is less than 100%.

The strength of the prepackaged enteral food feeding is reduced by diluting it with water. The enteral tube feeding formula determines the amount of water needed to dilute the prepackaged enteral food feeding to meet the strength ordered by the physician.

Before looking at the formula, it is important to understand following terms:

Concentration volume: This is the volume of the prepackaged enteral tube feeding, which is printed on the prepackage container.

Dilution factor: This is the strength specified by the physician's order and is given as a fraction or a percentage.

Total volume: This is the **total volume** of the enteral tube feeding after it has been diluted, which is the **concentration volume** and the added water.

Water to add: This is the amount of water you need to add to the prepackaged enteral food feeding to reach the total volume.

Calculating the amount of water to add to the prepackaged enteral food feeding is a two-step process.

1. Total volume = concentration volume/dilution factor
2. Water to add = total volume − concentration volume

Calculating Using The Enteral Tube Feeding Formula

Let's say that the physician ordered the patient to receive enteral food feeding of Jevity at 1/2 strength via a PEG tube at 80 mL/hr. You have on hand a 240-mL can of Jevity at 100% strength. How much water is needed to dilute the can of Jevity?

1. 480 mL = 240 mL/0.50

2. 240 mL = 480 mL − 240 mL

> **NURSING ALERT**
>
> Convert a fraction to a decimal by dividing the numerator (top number) by the denominator (bottom number). For example, 2/5 is converted by dividing 2 by 5. The remainder is the decimal equivalent, which is 0.40.
>
>   Convert a percentage to a decimal by dividing the percentage by 100. For example, 80%/100 = 0.80.

3. Enteral Tube Feeding Formula by Caloric Intake

Enteral tube feedings can also be ordered by calories rather than strength. The physician determines the number of calories the patient requires per day and prescribes prepackaged enteral food feeding. You must determine the amount of the prepackaged enteral food feeding to administer to the patient.

The prepackaged enteral food feeding label specifies the number of calories per volume. You use this information along with the physician's order to calculate the volume of the enteral food feeding to give to your patient.

Calculating Using the Enteral Tube Feeding Formula by Caloric Intake

Say the physician determined that the patient requires 2000 cal/day and orders that the patient receives Jevity as enteral tube feeding. The label on a can of Jevity states there are 300 cal in every 8 oz. You calculate the number of ounces of Jevity to administer to your patient by using the following formula:

1. Calories = calories/volume of prepackaged external tube feeding

2. Total number of ounces = calories ordered/calories/ounce

Let's apply the formula to the previous example:

1. 35 cal/oz = 280 cal/8 oz

2. 57 oz/day = 2000 cal per day/35 cal/oz

NURSING ALERT

Remember that 30 mL = 1 oz. You can convert ounces to milliliters if the volume you are administering is in milliliters.

CASE STUDY

CASE 1

Calculate the enteral tube feedings for the following orders.

QUESTION 1. The physician ordered 100 cc of 1/4 strength Sustacal via a PEG tube. On hand is a 240-cc can of Sustacal, which is at full strength. How much water is needed to dilute Sustacal?

QUESTION 2. The physician ordered 160 cc of 3/4 strength Enrich via a PEG tube. On hand is a 240-cc can of Enrich, which is at full strength. How much water is needed to dilute Enrich?

QUESTION 3. The physician ordered 280 cc of 1/2 strength Jevity via an NG tube. On hand is a 150-cc can of Jevity, which is at full strength. How much water is needed to dilute Jevity?

QUESTION 4. The physician ordered 240 cc of 3/4 strength Jevity via an NG tube. On hand is a 12-oz can of Jevity, which is at full strength. How much water is needed to dilute Jevity?

QUESTION 5. The physician ordered 80 cc of 1/4 strength Enrich via a PEG tube. On hand is a 240-mL can of Enrich, which is at full strength. How much water is needed to dilute Enrich?

QUESTION 6. The physician ordered 260 cc of 1/5 strength Sustacal via a PEG tube. On hand is a 300-cc can of Sustacal, which is at full strength. How much water is needed to dilute Sustacal?

QUESTION 7. The physician ordered 280 cc of 1/3 strength Jevity via an NG tube. On hand is a 350-cc can of Jevity, which is at 100% strength. How much water is needed to dilute Jevity?

QUESTION 8. The physician ordered 180 cc of 3/5 strength Enrich via a PEG tube. On hand is a 480-mL can of Enrich, which is at full strength. How much water is needed to dilute Enrich?

QUESTION 9. The physician ordered 140 cc of 2/5 strength Sustacal via a PEG tube. On hand is a 360-cc can of Sustacal, which is at full strength. How much water is needed to dilute Sustacal?

QUESTION 10. The physician ordered 220 cc of 4/5 strength Enrich via an NG tube. On hand is a 12-oz can of Enrich, which is at 100% strength. How much water is needed to dilute Enrich?

ANSWERS

1. 960 mL = 240 mL/0.25
   720 mL = 960 mL − 240 mL
2. 320 mL = 240 mL/0.75
   80 mL = 320 mL − 240 mL
3. 300 mL = 150 mL/0.5
   150 mL = 300 mL − 150 mL
4. 360 mL = 30 mL × 12 oz
   480 mL = 360 mL/0.75
   120 mL = 480 mL − 360 mL
5. 960 mL = 240 mL/0.25
   720 mL = 960 mL − 240 mL
6. 1500 mL = 300 mL/0.2
   1200 mL = 1500 mL − 300 mL
7. 1051 mL = 350 mL/0.333
   701 mL = 1051 mL − 350 mL
8. 800 mL = 480 mL/0.6
   320 mL = 800 mL − 480 mL
9. 900 mL = 360 mL/0.4
   540 mL = 900 mL − 360 mL
10. 360 mL = 30 mL × 12 oz
    450 mL = 360 mL/0.8
    90 mL = 450 mL − 360 mL

CASE STUDY

CASE 2

Calculate the enteral tube feedings by calories for the following orders.

QUESTION 1. The physician ordered that the patient receive 2500 cal/day. You have a 12-oz can of Sustacal. There are 250 cal in 8 oz of Sustacal. How many ounces of Sustacal will the patient receive each day?

QUESTION 2. The physician ordered that the patient receive 2000 cal/day. You have a 12-oz can of Jevity. There are 250 cal in 8 oz of Jevity. How many milliliters will the patient receive each day?

QUESTION 3. The physician ordered that the patient receive 2500 cal/day in 2-hour feedings. You have an 8-oz can of Jevity. There are 350 cal in 8 oz of Jevity. How many ounces will the patient receive in each feeding?

QUESTION 4. The physician ordered that the patient receive 2000 cal/day in 2-hour feedings. You have an 8-oz can of Enrich. There are 200 cal in 8 oz of Enrich. How many milliliters will the patient receive in each feeding?

QUESTION 5. The physician ordered that the patient receive 2500 cal/day in 4-hour feedings. You have a 240-mL can of Enrich. There are 250 cal in 8 oz of Enrich. How many milliliters will the patient receive in each day?

QUESTION 6. The physician ordered that the patient receive 3100 cal/day feedings in 2-hour feedings. You have a 240-mL can of Sustacal. There are 250 cal in 8 oz of Sustacal. How many calories will the patient receive in each feeding?

QUESTION 7. The physician ordered that the patient receive 1800 cal/day feedings. You have an 8-oz can of Sustacal. There are 150 cal in 8 oz of Sustacal. How many cans of Sustacal will the patient receive each day?

QUESTION 8. The physician ordered that the patient receive 2800 cal/day feedings. You have an 8-oz can of Enrich. There are 250 cal in 8 oz of Enrich. How many cans of Enrich will the patient receive each day?

QUESTION 9. The physician ordered that the patient receive 2500 cal/day feedings. You have a 12-oz can of Enrich. There are 150 cal in 8 oz of Enrich. How many cans of Enrich will the patient receive each day?

QUESTION 10. The physician ordered that the patient receive 3500 cal/day feedings in 2-hours feedings. You have a 12-oz can of Jevity. There are 250 cal in 8 oz of Jevity. How many cans of Jevity will the patient receive each day?

ANSWERS

1. 31.25 cal/oz = 250 cal/8 oz
   80 oz/day = 2500 cal/31.25 cal/oz
2. 31.25 cal/oz = 250 cal/8 oz
   64 oz = 2000 cal/31.25 cal/oz
   1920 mL/day = 64 oz × 30 mL
3. 43.75 cal/oz = 350 cal/8 oz
   57.1 oz/day = 2500 cal/43.75 cal/oz
   12 feedings/day = 24 hr/2 hr per feeding
   4.8 oz/feeding = 57.1 oz/day/12 feedings/day
4. 25 cal/oz = 200 cal/8 oz
   80 oz/day = 2000 cal/25 cal/oz
   12 feedings/day = 24 hr/2 hr per feeding
   6.7 oz/feeding = 80 oz/day/12 feedings/day
   201 mL/feeding = 6.7 oz/feeding × 30 mL
5. 31.25 cal/oz = 250 cal/8 oz
   80 oz/day = 2500 cal/31.25 cal/oz
   2400 mL/day = 80 oz × 30 mL
6. 12 feedings/day = 24 hr/2 hr per feeding
   258.3 cal/feeding = 3100 calories per day/12 feedings/day
7. 18.75 cal/oz = 150 cal/8 oz
   96 oz/day = 1800 cal/18.75 cal/oz
   12 cans per day = 96 oz/day/8 oz
8. 31.25 cal/oz = 250 cal/8 oz
   89.6 oz/day = 2800 cal/31.25 cal/oz
   11.2 cans per day = 89.6 oz/day/8 oz
9. 18.75 cal/oz = 150 cal/8 oz
   133.3 oz/day = 2500 cal/18.75 cal/oz
   11.1 cans per day = 133.3 oz/day/12 oz
10. 31.25 cal/oz = 250 cal/8 oz
    112 oz/day = 3500 cal/31.25 cal/oz
    9.3 cans per day = 112 oz/day/12 oz

1. The physician ordered that the patient receive 2100 cal/day. You have a 12-oz can of Jevity. There are 125 cal in 8 oz of Jevity. How many milliliters will the patient receive each day?

   A. 40.8 mL

   B. 403.8 mL

   C. 4032 mL

   D. 40.38 mL

2. The physician ordered 200 cc of 2/3 strength Jevity via a NG tube. On hand is a 250-cc can of Jevity, which is at 100% strength. How much water is needed to dilute Jevity?

   A. 231 mL

   B. 125 mL

   C. 312 mL

   D. 212 mL

3. The physician ordered 260 cc of 3/4 strength Enrich via a PEG tube. On hand is a 340-cc can of Enrich, which is at full strength. How much water is needed to dilute Enrich?

   A. 120 mL

   B. 119 mL

   C. 123 mL

   D. 113 mL

4. The physician ordered 240 cc of 2/5 strength Sustacal via a PEG tube. On hand is a 210-cc can of Sustacal, which is at full strength. How much water is needed to dilute Sustacal?

   A. 318 mL

   B. 314 mL

   C. 315 mL

   D. 300 mL

5. The physician ordered that the patient receive 3200 cal/day feedings in 2-hour feedings. You have a 240-mL can of Sustacal. There are 225 cal in 8 oz of Sustacal. How many calories will the patient receive in each feeding?

   A. 266.7 cal/feeding

   B. 26.67 cal/feeding

   C. 2.6 cal/feeding

   D. 66.7 cal/feeding

6. The physician ordered 280 cc of 1/4 strength Enrich via a PEG tube. On hand is a 140-mL can of Enrich, which is at full strength. How much water is needed to dilute Enrich?

   A. 420 mL
   B. 400 mL
   C. 415 mL
   D. 404 mL

7. The physician ordered 360 cc of 4/5 strength Enrich via a PEG tube. On hand is a 280-cc can of Enrich, which is at full strength. How much water is needed to dilute Enrich?

   A. 69 mL
   B. 75 mL
   C. 70 mL
   D. 74 mL

8. The physician ordered that the patient receive 2000 calories/day. You have a 12-oz can of Enrich. There are 275 cal in 8 oz of Enrich. How many cans of Enrich will the patient receive each day?

   A. 4.8 cans
   B. 4.7 cans
   C. 4 cans
   D. 4.9 cans

9. The physician ordered 100 cc of 1/5 strength Sustacal via a PEG tube. On hand is a 120-cc can of Sustacal, which is at full strength. How much water is needed to dilute Sustacal?

   A. 450 mL
   B. 480 mL
   C. 400 ml
   D. 350 mL

10. The physician ordered that the patient receive 2200 cal/day. You have a 12-oz can of Sustacal. There are 220 cal in 8 oz of Sustacal. How many cans of Sustacal will the patient receive each day?

    A. 6 cans/day
    B. 6.9 cans/day
    C. 6.6 cans/day
    D. 6.7 cans/day

CORRECT ANSWERS AND RATIONALES

1. C. 4032 mL
2. B. 125 mL
3. D. 113 mL
4. C. 315 mL
5. A. 266.7 cal/feeding
6. A. 420 mL
7. C. 70 mL
8. A. 4.8 cans
9. B. 480 mL
10. D. 6.7 cans/day

Part II

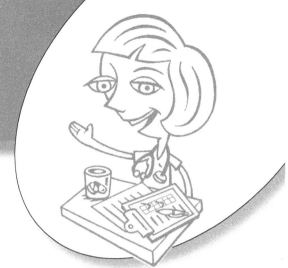

Basic Math Skills

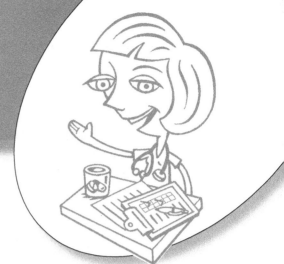

Positive and Negative Numbers

LEARNING OBJECTIVES

1. Understanding Positive and Negative Numbers
2. The Rules of Signs

1. Understanding Positive and Negative Numbers

Positive and negative numbers can be challenging to understand because positive numbers are typically used in everyday calculations. A positive number is a value that is greater than zero. Technically, a plus sign (+) is placed in front of a positive number to indicate that the number is positive; however, it has become common practice not to use the plus sign unless negative number is used. Therefore, no sign in front of the number means the number is a positive number.

A negative number is a value that is less than zero. A minus sign (−) is always placed in front of a negative number to indicate that the number is less than zero. If the minus sign is missing, then the presumption is the value is a positive number.

The best way to visual positive and negative numbers is to draw a line (Figure 10–1). Mark the center of the line 0. Insert positive numbers beginning with 1 to the right of the zero and insert negative numbers beginning with −1 to the left of the zero. There should be equal spaces between numbers.

> **NURSING ALERT**
>
> Think of the line as a scale of a thermometer that measures temperature above and below zero.

Clarifying the Confusion of Positive and Negative Numbers

Positive and negative numbers can become challenging to understand, particularly the relative size of the negative numbers. You know that the number 3 is greater than the number 1. Notice that there is no sign; therefore, these are positive numbers.

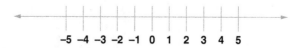

FIGURE 10–1 • Positive numbers are greater than zero and negative numbers are less than zero.

However, the number −3 is smaller than number −1. Strange as this sounds, it is true. Let's take another look at the line in Figure 10–1 to understand the relative size of negative numbers.

In the center of the line is zero. Zero means there is no value. Numbers increase in size going to the right of zero. Numbers become bigger and bigger compared with the number to the left. That is 5 is greater than 3.

Let's reverse the count. Start with 5 and count backwards to zero. Each number is smaller than the previous number. Don't stop at zero. Continue counting backwards. The numbers continue to become smaller than the previous number. Therefore, −3 is smaller than −1. Remember this process when using positive and negative numbers.

2. The Rules of Signs

Numbers in an addition or subtraction are either positive or negative. A positive number is preceded by a plus sign (+) and a negative number is preceded by a negative (−) sign. Typically, the plus sign is not used when writing a positive number. If you don't see a sign, then presume that the number is a positive number.

Use parenthesis when writing the sign of the number such as (+3) or (−3). The parenthesis helps to visually separate the sign and number from the addition sign and minus sign.

When two numbers are added or subtracted, the sign of the operation (add [+] or subtract [−]) and the second number determines the sign of the results of the calculation. Here are the rules of signs (Table 10–1).

Adding and Subtracting Negative Numbers

Adding two numbers is probably not new to you such as 3 + 2. In order to better understand positive and negative numbers, let's place a plus sign in front of each number since these numbers are all positive numbers. Rewrite the expression as: (+3) + (+2) =

TABLE 10–1 The Sign of Each Number in the Calculation Determines the Sign of the Resulting Number	
Signs	**Results**
Two like signs	Positive (+)
Two unlike signs	Negative (−)

Now apply the rules of signs. The addition sign (+) and the positive 2 (+2) are both positive signs. Therefore, the sign does not change and the result is a positive number. (+3) + (+2) = (+5).

Subtracting a negative value is the same as adding that value. Let's change the calculation to (+6) − (−3). There are two like signs, minus (−) and a negative (−) 3. Since there are two like signs, replace them with a positive sign and rewrite the expression as 6 + 3, then perform the operation. The result is a positive 9.

Adding a negative value or subtracting a positive value is subtraction. Take for example (+6) − (+3). The signs are different (minus and plus); therefore, the expression is rewritten as 6 − 3 = 3.

The same process is performed if a negative number is added to a positive number as shown in this example: (+5) + (−8). The signs are different (plus and minus); therefore, the expression is rewritten as 5 − 8 = (−3).

Multiplying Positive and Negative Numbers

Multiplying positive and negative numbers is a two-step process. The first step is to carryout multiplication ignoring the positive and negative signs. The second step is to determine the sign of the result. When multiplying positive and negative numbers, determine the sign of the results based on the signs used in the expression (see Table 10–2).

Let's take a simple example of 4 × 5. The first step is to multiply the expression. The result is 20. The next step is to determine the sign of the result. Since both are positive numbers, the result is also positive; therefore, 4 × 5 = 20.

Now let's change both numbers to negative numbers by writing (−4) × (−5). Follow the same process to calculate this expression, 4 × 5 = 20. Next determine the sign of the result. Since both numbers are negative, the sign of the result is positive; therefore, (−4) × (−5) = 20.

TABLE 10–2 Determine the Sign of the Result by Comparing Signs in the Expression as Shown in This Table	
Signs	**Results**
Positive × Positive	Positive (+)
Negative × Negative	Positive (+)
Positive × Negative	Negative (−)
Negative × Positive	Negative (−)

Multiplying an expression with positive and negative numbers may appear challenging but following the rules makes the calculation straightforward to perform. Try this expression: $(-4) \times 5$. First, perform the multiplication, $4 \times 5 = 20$. Next, determine the sign of the result. These numbers have different signs; therefore, the result is negative: $(-4) \times 5 = (-20)$.

The same result is true when multiplying positive and negative numbers such as $4 \times (-5) = -20$.

Dividing Positive and Negative Numbers

Dividing positive and negative numbers is a two-step process very similar to multiplying positive and negative numbers. The first step is to carryout division ignoring the positive and negative signs. The second step is to determine the sign of the result. When dividing positive and negative numbers, determine the sign of the result based on the signs used in the expression (see Table 10–3).

Try this example of $10 \div 5$. The first step is to divide the expression. The result is 2. The next determine the sign of the result. Since both are positive numbers, the result is also positive; therefore, $10 \div 5 = 2$.

Change both numbers to negative numbers by writing $(-10) \div (-5)$. Follow the same process by performing the division first, $10 \div 5 = 2$. Next determine the sign of the result. Both numbers are negative; therefore, the sign of the result is positive: $(-10) \div (-5) = 2$.

Dividing an expression with positive and negative numbers is also similar to multiplication. Try this expression: $(-10) \div 5$. First, divide $10 \div 5 = 2$. Then, determine the sign of the result. These numbers have different signs; therefore, the result is negative: $(-10) \div 5 = (-2)$.

The same result is true when dividing positive and negative numbers such as $10 \div (-5) = (-2)$.

TABLE 10–3 Here Are the Rules to Follow When Dividing Positive and Negative Numbers	
Signs	Results
Positive ÷ Positive	Positive (+)
Negative ÷ Negative	Positive (+)
Positive ÷ Negative	Negative (−)
Negative ÷ Positive	Negative (−)

CASE STUDY

CASE 1
Calculate the following positive and negative numbers.

QUESTION 1. $(-5) \times (-7) =$

QUESTION 2. $10 \div (-3) =$

QUESTION 3. $(-8) + 4 =$

QUESTION 4. $9 - (-4) =$

QUESTION 5. $(-6) \times (-2) =$

QUESTION 6. $(-6) \div (-2) =$

QUESTION 7. $(-5) + 7 =$

QUESTION 8. $5 - (-8) =$

QUESTION 9. $(-4) \div 2 =$

QUESTION 10. $8 + (-6) =$

ANSWERS

1. $(-5) \times (-7) = 35$
2. $10 \div (-3) = (-3.33)$
3. $(-8) + 4 = (-4)$
4. $9 - (-4) = 13$
5. $(-6) \times (-2) = 12$
6. $(-6) \div (-2) = 3$
7. $(-5) + 7 = 2$
8. $5 - (-8) = 13$
9. $(-4) \div 2 = (-2)$
10. $8 + (-6) = 2$

FINAL CHECK-UP

1. The children's unit at the hospital encourages young patients to eat meals by awarding points that can be redeemed once a day for a prize. Failure to eat meals causes the young patient to lose points. Six-year-old Bob received 10 points before lunch. He told the nurse that he ate all his lunch. The nurse awarded Bob 5 points, bringing Bob's total to 15 points. However, the certified nursing assistant (CNA) told the nurse Bob did not eat all his lunch. The nurse deducted points using the following expression: $15 - (+5)$. This states that a positive 5 points is being removed from the total points. What is the result of this expression?

   A. 15
   B. 20
   C. 10
   D. 5

2. A patient who is recovering from a stroke undergoes physical therapy to help regain his ability to ambulate. The therapist measures the number of footsteps the patient takes regardless of the direction. In each of the three attempts, the patient took four steps backwards. The therapist recorded this as $(-4) \times 3$. How many steps did the patient take?

   A. (−4 steps)
   B. 4 steps
   C. (−13 steps)
   D. (−12 steps)

3. A patient with liver failure underwent paracentesis for ascites. Each day 2 L of fluid are removed. How many liters were removed in the past 3 days?

   A. 5 L
   B. 1.3 L
   C. 6 L
   D. 1.5 L

4. A patient was brought into the emergency department after exposure to extremely cold weather when he fell through the ice in a frozen pond. The temperature dropped from 15°F to −5°F. How many degrees did this drop?

   A. 15°F
   B. 20°F
   C. 10°F
   D. (−10°F)

5. A patient who had knee surgery was placed on a continuous passive motion (CPM) device that mechanically manipulates the patient's leg. The fully extended leg is measured as 0 degrees. The CPM device bends the knee measured as less than 0 degrees, which is a negative number. At the beginning of the week, the patient knee moved −5 degrees. At the end of the week, the patient was able to move his knee −14 degrees. What distance has the knee moved over the week?

   A. 9 degrees
   B. 19 degrees
   C. (−19 degrees)
   D. (−9 degrees)

6. The nurse is pouring 2 oz of juice for each patient from a 24-oz container of juice. The nurse has six patients. How many oz are removed from the container?

   A. (−24 oz)
   B. 2 oz
   C. 6 oz
   D. (−12 oz)

7. A patient was given range of motion exercise for her arm. Holding her arm straight in front of her is considered 0 degrees. Raising her arm is considered positive degrees and lowering her arm is considered negative degrees. She lowered her arm 5 degrees on Monday and 10 degrees on Tuesday. How many degrees in total did she move her arm?

   A. 5 degrees
   B. (−15 degrees)
   C. (−5 degrees)
   D. (−10 degrees)

8. By Friday, the patient in question 7 was able to lower her arm 32 degrees. How much movement since Monday she did?

   a. (−37 degrees)
   b. 37 degrees
   c. (−27 degrees)
   d. (−10 degrees)

9. A patient with liver failure underwent paracentesis for ascites. Over the past 4 days 9 L of fluid are removed. About how many liters were removed a day?

   A. 2.25 L
   B. (−2.25 L)
   C. 2 L
   D. (−2 L)

10. A patient's blood pressure was very high. You administered medication to reduce the patient's blood pressure. The patient's systolic blood pressure decreased 2 mm Hg every hour for 4 hours. How much did the patient's systolic blood pressure decrease?

A. (−8 mm Hg)

B. (−4 mm Hg)

C. 4 mm Hg

D. (−1 mm Hg)

CORRECT ANSWERS AND RATIONALES

1. C. 10; Hint: Unlike signs is a negative.
2. D. (−12 steps); Hint: Unlike signs
3. C. 6 L; Hint: (−2 L/day) × (−3 days) = 6 L (Negative signs are used to represent the past. Like signs result in a positive sign.)
4. B. 20°F; Hint: 15°F − (−5°F) Like signs result in a positive sign.
5. D. (−9 degrees); Hint: (−14 degrees) − (−5 degrees) Like signs result in a positive sign (−14 degrees) + 5.
6. D. (−12 oz); Hint: 6 patients × (−2 oz) = (−12 oz) Unlike signs result in a negative sign.
7. B. (−15 degrees); Hint: (−10 degrees) + (−5 degrees) = (−15 degrees)
8. C. (−27 degrees); Hint: (−32 degrees) − (−5 degrees) = (−27 degrees)
9. A. 2.25 L; Hint: (−9 Liters) ÷ (−4 days) = 2.25 liters
10. A. (−8 mm Hg); Hint: 4 hr × (−2 mm Hg) = −8 mm Hg Unlike numbers result in a negative number.

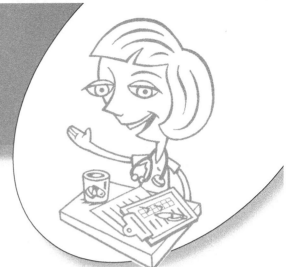

chapter **11**

Fractions, Decimals, and Percentage

1. Understanding Fractions

A fraction is part of a whole of something. For example, each part of a tablet that is split in half is a fraction of the whole tablet. The whole is written as 1 such as 1 tablet. Each part of the whole is written as less than one as a fraction.

A fraction is written as two numbers separated by an angled line commonly referred to as a forward slash. The top number is called the numerator and the bottom number is called the denominator. The top number (numerator) is the number that represents the part of the whole, and the bottom number (denominator) is the number that represents the number of parts that make up the whole (Figure 11–1).

> **NURSING ALERT**
>
> If there is no part of the whole (fraction), then the top number (numerator) and the bottom number (denominator) are the same numbers such as 10/10. You can say this is 10 parts of 10, which is really the whole—no fraction.

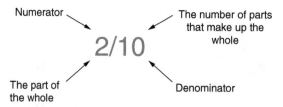

FIGURE 11–1 • This fraction tells you that you have 1 part of a whole thing that is made up of 2 parts such as a tablet that you split in half.

Number of parts of the whole

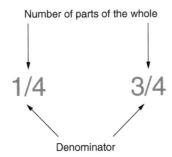

Denominator

FIGURE 11.2 • Comparing two fractions that have the same denominator is a straightforward process because the denominators are the same.

Comparing Fractions

There are times when you are presented with two fractions and need to know if they are equal or more or less than the other. Sometimes the comparison is easy to do because the denominator of each fraction is the same.

Figure 11–2 shows two fractions—1/4 and 3/4. The bottom number of each tells you there are four parts that make up the whole. One fraction represents 1 part and the other 3 parts. Therefore, you know 3 is greater than 1 and therefore 3/4 is greater than 1/4.

Comparing Fractions That Have Different Denominators

Comparing fractions that have different denominators can be a challenge because each has a different denominator. This means each fraction has a different number of parts that make up the whole as seen in Figure 11–3 where one fraction is 1/4 and the other is 2/5.

Let's explore what these fractions are telling us. The fraction 1/4 is saying that 4 parts make up the whole and this fraction is one of those parts. This is like breaking a tablet into four pieces and holding one of those pieces in your hand.

The fraction 2/5 is saying 5 parts make up the whole and the fraction contains two of those parts. This is like breaking a tablet into five pieces and holding two of those pieces in your hand. You need to have the same denominator before comparing these fractions. To do this, you need to find the smallest number that can be divided by both denominators. This is called the lowest common denominator. The easiest way to do this is to use a multiplication table (Table 11–1).

What number can be evenly divided by both denominators 4 and 5? Find where column 4 and row 5 merge and you'll notice the value 20. This means

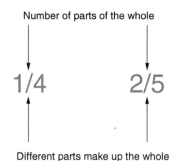

Number of parts of the whole

1/4   2/5

Different parts make up the whole

FIGURE 11–3 • Fractions that have unlike denominators require you to convert the denominators before comparing fractions.

that both 4 and 5 can be evenly divided into 20. Likewise, you could find where column 5 and row 4 merge and you'll also see 20. Number 20 is a likely candidate as the lowest common denominator.

Next, you need to convert the denominator of both fractions to 20. That is, you want to write that the whole consists of 20 parts instead of either 4 parts (1/4) or 5 parts (1/5).

You convert the fractions by multiplying the numerator and the denominator by the other fraction's denominator as shown in Figure 11–4. Now both fractions define the whole as having 20 parts. The numerators of each fraction were adjusted to reflect the new denominator. You can now easily compare the number of parts represented by each fraction.

TABLE 11–1   A Multiplication Table Can Help Identify the Lowest Common Denominator

	1	2	3	4	5	6	7	8	9	10	11	12
1	1	2	3	4	5	6	7	8	9	10	11	12
2	2	4	6	8	10	12	14	16	18	20	22	24
3	3	6	9	12	15	18	21	24	27	30	33	36
4	8	8	12	16	20	24	28	32	36	40	44	48
5	5	10	15	20	25	30	35	40	45	50	55	60
6	6	12	18	24	30	36	42	48	54	60	66	72
7	7	14	21	28	35	42	49	56	63	70	77	84
8	8	16	24	32	40	48	56	64	72	80	88	96
9	9	18	27	36	45	54	63	72	81	90	99	108
10	10	20	30	40	50	60	70	80	90	100	110	120
11	11	22	33	44	55	66	77	88	99	110	121	132
12	12	24	36	48	60	72	84	96	108	120	132	144

$$\frac{1 \times 5 = 5}{4 \times 5 = 20}$$

$$\frac{2 \times 4 = 8}{5 \times 4 = 20}$$

FIGURE 11−4 • Multiply numerators and denominators to convert fractions to the lowest common denominator.

Adding Fractions

Two or more fractions can be added to form another fraction. Let's say you have pitcher that holds 4 qt of fluid. The pitcher currently holds 2 qt of fluid and is therefore 2/4 full, which is half full. You add 1 quarter of fluid to the pitcher (1/4). Adding these fractions together will give you 3/4 full.

Figure 11–5 shows how to add fractions. The first fraction is saying there are 2 parts of a whole that has 4 parts. The second fraction is saying there is 1 part of a whole that has 4 parts. Since the number of parts in the whole (denominator) is the same in each fraction, all that is needed is to add together the numerators. The result is a fraction that is saying there are 3 parts of a whole that has 4 parts.

> **NURSING ALERT**
>
> Each fraction must have a common denominator. If there are different denominators, then you must convert each fraction to a common denominator before adding the fractions.

Subtracting Fractions

A fraction can be subtracted from another fraction. Let's return to the pitcher of fluid. The pitcher can hold four quarters and currently holds three quarters. We could pour 1 qt from the pitcher, which is subtracting.

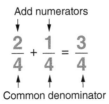

Add numerators

$$\frac{2}{4} + \frac{1}{4} = \frac{3}{4}$$

Common denominator

FIGURE 11−5 • Numerators can be added together as long as fractions have the same common denominator.

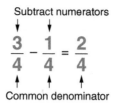

Subtract numerators

$$\frac{3}{4} - \frac{1}{4} = \frac{2}{4}$$

Common denominator

FIGURE 11.6 • Numerators can be subtracted as long as fractions have the same common denominator.

Figure 11–6 illustrates how to subtract fractions. The first fraction is saying there are 3 parts to a whole that has 4 parts. The second fraction is saying there is 1 part of a whole what has 4 parts. The whole could be the pitcher of fluid.

Only the numerators are subtracted. The denominators are carried over the answer. All fractions must have the same denominator before subtracting values.

Multiplying Fractions

Fractions are multiplied by multiplying both numerators and both denominators of each fraction. Figure 11–7 shows how to multiple 3/4 by 1/5. Notice that you don't need a common denominator to multiply fractions.

In this example, the numerators 3 times 1 equal 3 and the denominators 4 times 5 equal 20. The result is 3/20.

> **NURSING ALERT**
>
> Multiplying fractions always results in a smaller fraction, which is different from multiplying whole numbers that results in a larger number.

Dividing Fractions

Fractions are divided by using the reciprocal of the second fraction. The reciprocal of the second fraction is obtained by flipping the second fraction. Let's say the second fraction is 2/3 as illustrated in Figure 11–8. The reciprocal is

Multiply numerators

$$\frac{3}{4} \times \frac{1}{5} = \frac{3}{20}$$

Multiply denominator

FIGURE 11–7 • Multiply two fractions by multiplying numerators and denominators of those fractions.

$$\frac{3}{5} \div \frac{2}{3} =$$

Flip the second fraction

Multiply numerators ⟶

Multiply denominator ⟶

$$\frac{3}{5} \times \frac{3}{2} = \frac{9}{10}$$

FIGURE 11−8 • When dividing two fractions, flip the second fraction to create the reciprocal, then multiply the fractions.

3/2—the numerator becomes the denominator and the denominator becomes the numerator.

Dividing fractions is a two-step process. The first step is to flip the second fraction. The final step is to multiply the numerators and multiply the denominators just as if you are multiplying fractions.

In Figure 11–8, 3/5 is being divided by 2/3. 2/3 is flipped to create the reciprocal, which is 3/2 and then the numerators and the denominators are multiplied resulting in 9/10.

Improper Fractions

An improper fraction is a fraction where the numerator is larger than the denominator as shown in Figure 11–9. An improper fraction is saying the same as a proper fraction.

The numerator represents the number of pieces of the whole. The denominator represents the number of pieces that make up the whole. Figure 11–9 shows the fraction 5/2. The number of pieces of the whole represented by the numerator is 5. The number of pieces that make up the whole is 2.

Since the 5 pieces (numerator) is more than the number of pieces that make up the whole (2), the improper fraction represents more than the whole. A proper fraction represents less than the whole because the numerator is less than the denominator.

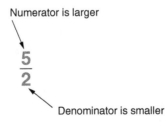

Numerator is larger

$$\frac{5}{2}$$

Denominator is smaller

FIGURE 11.9 • An improper fraction is a fraction where the numerator is larger than the denominator.

$$\frac{4 \div 4 = 1}{8 \div 4 = 4}$$

Simple fraction

FIGURE 11–10 • A proper fraction can be reduced to a simple fraction by reducing the fraction to lowest terms.

An improper fraction can be converted into a mixed number. A mixed number consists of a whole number and a fraction. An improper fraction is converted by dividing the numerator by the denominator such as 5 ÷ 2. The result is 2.5. In other words, the improper fraction represents two whole numbers and a fraction of a whole. The fraction of the whole number is represented as a decimal value (see Chapter 12). This result shows 0.5 decimal value that converts to 1/2 fraction (see Fractions and Decimals).

Therefore, the improper fraction 5/2 is saying there are 2 whole numbers and 1/2 of a whole number.

Reducing Fractions

A proper fraction can be reduced to a simple fraction by reducing a fraction to lowest terms. A simple fraction is a fraction that cannot be reduced. For example, 4/8 is a proper fraction but not a simple fraction because 4/8 can be reduced to lower terms.

Reducing a fraction requires the use of a greatest common factor (GCF) of the numerator and the denominator of the fraction. The greatest common factor is the largest number that can be divided evenly into both the numerator and the denominator.

The greatest common factor in the fraction 4/8 is 4 (see Figure 11–10). That is, 4 can be evenly divided into both the numerator and the denominator. The result is the simple fraction 1/4. 1/4 cannot be reduced to lower terms.

2. Fractions and Decimals

A decimal is a part of a whole of something and another way to write a fraction. A decimal is less than 1 (whole) and more than 0. A decimal value is written by a number that is preceded by a period. The period is called a decimal point. Numbers to the left of the decimal point represent whole things. Numbers to the right of the decimal point represent part of the whole thing (see Figure 11–11).

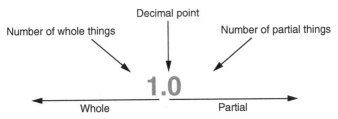

FIGURE 11–11 • Values to the left of the decimal point are whole numbers and values to the right of the decimal point are partial numbers.

Let's say you have a tablet. The tablet is a whole thing. You could write "1 tablet" or write "1.0 tablet" because both tell you the same. Both represent 1 tablet. "1 tablet" implies there is no partial value (i.e., no decimal value). "1.0 tablet" explicitly tells you there is no partial value because the 1 to the left of the decimal point means 1 whole thing and the 0 to the left of the decimal point means there are zero parts of the thing.

Fractions and decimals are related because each is used to write a partial value. Let's take a closer look at this relationship by splitting a tablet in half (see Figure 11–12). The whole tablet can be written a 1 or as a fraction as 1/1. Remember from Section 1 of this chapter that the top number in a fraction is called the numerator and indicates the number of parts of the whole that is represented in the fraction. The bottom number is called the denominator, which indicates the number that is the whole. Therefore, 1/1 is saying that there is 1 part and 1 whole, which is another way of saying 1. That is, the fraction represents 1 part of something that has 1 part (i.e., the whole thing).

The way to represent the 1 tablet as a decimal is by writing 1.0. The 1 is to the left of the decimal meaning the number is a whole thing. Since the number is 1, then we know there is only 1 whole thing. A 0 is to the right of the decimal. Numbers to the left of the decimal represent part of the whole thing. In this example, there isn't any part because the number is 0.

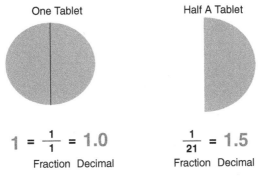

FIGURE 11–12 • A fraction or a decimal can be used to write 1 tablet or part of a tablet.

When you split a tablet in half, a half of tablet is less than the whole tablet. The half can be written as a fraction 1/2 indicating this is 1 part of a whole that has 2 parts. You write the half tablet as a decimal as 0.5.

NURSING ALERT

A fraction implies division. Think of the line in the fraction as a division symbol telling you to divide the numerator (top number) by the denominator (bottom number). In the fraction 1/2, we're told to divide 1 by 2. The result of the division is a decimal value of 0.5.

Adding Decimals

Adding decimals is very similar to adding whole numbers with a few exceptions. First, write the numbers so that the decimals are aligned (see Figure 11–13). Next carry the decimal to result and perform the addition as shown in Figure 11–13 where 0.5 + 0.3 = 0.8. Make sure that you place a 0 to the left of the decimal if there isn't a whole number. This helps you see the decimal point.

A number can be a mixed number, which is a mix of a whole number and decimal number. Stack the numbers aligning the decimals as shown in Figure 11–14, then add the numbers. The first example in Figure 11–14 is 1.5 + 0.3, the result is 1.8.

The second example is a little different because the sum of the decimal values equals 1. That is, adding 0.5 (half) and 0.5 (half) is 1. The decimal values are greater than 1 so you carryover the remaining value and add the number to the left column of numbers.

The third example in Figure 11–14 presents another variation of decimal values that you will likely encounter. In this example, you are adding 1.5 + 0.53.

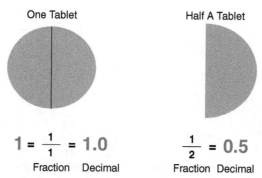

$$1 = \frac{1}{1} = 1.0 \qquad \frac{1}{2} = 0.5$$

Fraction Decimal   Fraction Decimal

FIGURE 11–13 • Line up the decimal points before adding numbers that have a decimal.

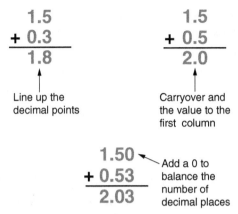

$$\begin{array}{r} 1.5 \\ +\ 0.3 \\ \hline 1.8 \end{array}$$

↑

Line up the
decimal points

$$\begin{array}{r} 1.5 \\ +\ 0.5 \\ \hline 2.0 \end{array}$$

↑

Carryover and
the value to the
first column

$$\begin{array}{r} 1.50 \\ +\ 0.53 \\ \hline 2.03 \end{array}$$

Add a 0 to
balance the
number of
decimal places

FIGURE 11–14 • Line up the decimals in mixed numbers, then add the numbers making sure to carryover the value to the whole number if decimal values 1 or greater.

Notice that 0.53 has two decimal places and 1.5 has one decimal place. Follow the same steps to setup the numbers as if both numbers had the same number of decimal places. However, it is best to add a 0 at the end of the 1.5 to balance the number of decimal places. Adding 0 after a decimal doesn't change the value of the number.

Subtracting Decimals

Subtracting decimals is very similar to subtracting whole numbers and adding decimals. Figure 11–15 shows three examples of subtracting decimals. First, line up the decimals as you do when adding decimals. Next, bring down the decimals point and perform subtraction.

$$\begin{array}{r} 1.5 \\ -\ 0.3 \\ \hline 1.2 \end{array}$$

↑

Line up the
decimal points

$$\begin{array}{r} 1.5 \\ -\ 0.5 \\ \hline 1.0 \end{array}$$

$$\begin{array}{r} 1.50 \\ -\ 0.53 \\ \hline 0.97 \end{array}$$

Add a 0 to
balance the
number of
decimal places

FIGURE 11–15 • Line up the decimal points, then follow the same process that you use to subtract whole numbers.

Notice the third example, 1.5 − .53. A 0 was added to the end of the 1.5 to balance the decimal places. This makes it easier to visualize the calculation. The 0 is less than 3; therefore, you need to take 1 from the next left column just as you normally do in subtraction. You also need to carryover 1 from the whole number to the first decimal number before subtracting. This too is the same process as you do when subtracting whole numbers.

Multiplying Decimals

Multiplying decimals is very similar to multiplying whole number except you must carefully place the decimal point in the result. Multiplying decimals is a two-step process. The first step is multiplication and the second step is positioning the decimal point properly in the result.

Let's see how to multiple 1.5×2 as shown in Figure 11−16. Setup the multiplication problem by aligning each number to the right regardless of the position of the decimal point, which is different from addition and subtraction of decimals. Next multiply 2×15 (notice that the decimal is ignored). The result is 30. The final step is to position the decimal point in the result.

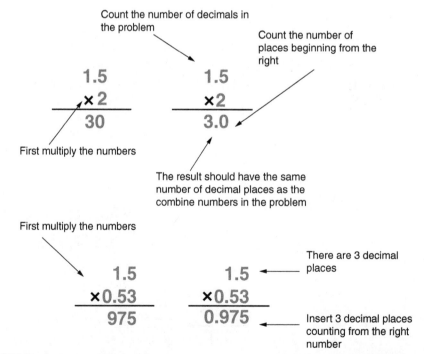

FIGURE 11−16 • Align both numbers to the right, then multiply the numbers. Count the number of decimal places in both numbers and insert the same number of decimal places into the result.

Here's how to do it. Count the number of decimal points in both numbers. The top number is 1.5 and there is one decimal point. The bottom number is 2, a whole number, and does not have any decimal point. Therefore, the total number of decimal points in the multiplication problem is one.

Start counting from before the right digit in the result and stop when you reach the number of decimal points in the multiplication problem and insert the decimal point in the result. In the first example in Figure 11–16, the decimal point is placed between the 3 and the 0 making the result 3.0.

The second example in Figure 11–16 shows multiplication of two numbers each having a decimal point. Follow the same procedure to solve this problem. First perform multiplication. Count the number of decimal places in both numbers, which is three and insert the decimal point three positions from the right in the result.

Dividing Decimals

Dividing decimals is also very similar to dividing whole number except you must position the decimal point in the proper place in the result. The first example in Figure 11–17 shows a mixed number (1.5) being divided by a

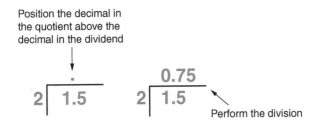

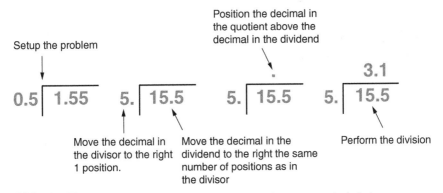

FIGURE 11–17 • Move decimal places in the dividend the same number of places you move the decimal point in the divisor.

whole number. Since there is one decimal place in this problem, insert the decimal point about the existing decimal point and then perform division.

Dividing a decimal value by another decimal value such as the second example in Figure 11–17 requires another step. First, step up the division problem. Next, adjust the position of the decimal place. You do this by moving the decimal point of the dividend to the right the same number of decimal places there are in the divisor.

The dividend is 1.55 and the divisor is 0.5. The divisor has one decimal place. Move the decimal in the dividend one place to the right (15.5). Also move the decimal place of the divisor one decimal place to the right (5). Insert the decimal place in the quotient above the decimal place in the dividend. Finally, perform the division.

3. Percentage

A percentage is another way of writing a partial value just like using a decimal and a fraction. A percent means per hundred or a value out of a 100 values. This may sound confusing but think of 100 as one whole thing and a value less than a 100 as less than a whole thing.

Use the percentage symbol (%) after the number to indicate that the number represents a percentage rather than an actual number. For example, 100% means the same as 1.0 and 1/1 and 1. Let's look at the smallest whole percent, which is 1%. It is the same as 0.01 and 1/100.

Converting to a Percentage

Any fraction or decimal can be converted to a percentage by multiplying by 100 as illustrated in Figure 11–18. Let's say that a whole was divided into 5 parts, that is, 1/5. Remember that a fraction is another statement of division. That is, 1 divided by 5, which is 0.2. Convert 0.2 to a percentage by multiplying 0.2 × 100, which equals 20%.

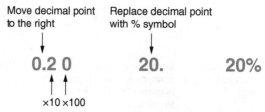

FIGURE 11–18 • Convert a decimal value to a percentage by multiplying the decimal value by 100.

> ### NURSING ALERT
>
> A more efficient way to multiply and divide a decimal is by moving the decimal point to the right or left as shown in Figure 11–19. Moving the decimal place to the right is the same as multiplication. Moving the decimal point to the left is the same as division. The first decimal place represents 10; the second decimal place represents 100; and the third decimal place represents 1000.

Determine the Value of a Percentage

Percentages can be used to determine the part of the whole such as 50% of a 650 mg tablet. 650 mg is 100%. Half of 100% is 50%. However, you want to know what is half of 650 mg. Here are the steps to follow:

1. Convert 50% to a decimal by replacing the % symbol with a decimal (50.) then divide 50. by 100. Remember that division is performed by moving the decimal point to the left. One place to the left is like dividing by 10. Two places to the left are like dividing by 100. Therefore, 50% is equal to 0.5 decimal value.

2. Multiply 650 mg by 0.5. = 325 mg (see Multiplying Decimals).

Half of the whole 650 mg tablet is 325 mg.

Determine the Percentage of a Value

There'll be occasions when you'll know the whole and the part and need to calculate the percentage of the part of the whole. Let's say there are three units that can have a collective census of 200 patients. Currently there are 56 patients on these units. What percentage is 56 patients of 200 patients?

Here's how to calculate the percentage:

1. Divide 56 by 200. The result is 0.28.

2. Multiply 0.28 by 100 to arrive at the percentage. Remember that multiplication is the same as moving the decimal point to the right. One place is 10 and two places is 100. Therefore, you move the decimal point to the right two places. The result is 28%. That is, 56 patients are 28% of 200 patients.

Move decimal point to the left to divide   Move decimal point to the right to multiple
⟵ _____   _____ ⟶

0.20

FIGURE 11–19 • Move the decimal to the right to multiply and to the left to divide the decimal value.

CASE STUDY

CASE 1
Calculate the following fractions.

QUESTION 1. $2/5 \times 3/4 =$

QUESTION 2. $4/6 + 2/7 =$

QUESTION 3. $4/9 \div 4/5 =$

QUESTION 4. $2/6 - 1/4 =$

QUESTION 5. $3/7 \times 1/2 =$

QUESTION 6. $1/8 \div 2/5 =$

QUESTION 7. $1/3 + 1/2 =$

QUESTION 8. $5/7 \times 3/4 =$

QUESTION 9. $3/8 \div 4/5 =$

QUESTION 10. $1/8 + 4/8 =$

ANSWERS

1. $2/5 \times 3/4 = 3/10$
2. $4/6 + 2/7 = 20/21$
3. $4/9 \div 4/5 = 5/9$
4. $2/6 - 1/4 = 1/12$
5. $3/7 \times 1/2 = 3/14$
6. $1/8 \div 2/5 = 5/16$
7. $1/3 + 1/2 = 5/6$
8. $5/7 \times 3/4 = 15/28$
9. $3/8 \div 4/5 = 15/32$
10. $1/8 + 4/8 = 5/8$

CASE STUDY

CASE 2
Calculate the following decimals.

QUESTION 1. $0.15 \div 0.5 =$

QUESTION 2. $7 \times 1.35 =$

QUESTION 3. $0.8 + 3.5 =$

QUESTION 4. $0.56 - 0.34 =$

QUESTION 5. $6 \times 0.87 =$

QUESTION 6. $1.88 \div 0.4 =$

QUESTION 7. $0.45 + 2.33 =$

QUESTION 8. $0.23 \times 0.12 =$

QUESTION 9. $0.125 \div 2 =$

QUESTION 10. $0.025 + 1.75 =$

ANSWERS

1. $0.15 \div 0.5 = 0.3$
2. $7 \times 1.35 = 9.45$
3. $0.8 + 3.5 = 4.3$
4. $0.56 - 0.34 = 0.22$
5. $6 \times 0.87 = 5.22$
6. $1.88 \div 0.4 = 4.7$
7. $0.45 + 2.33 = 2.78$
8. $0.23 \times 0.12 = 0.276$
9. $0.125 \div 2 = 0.0625$
10. $0.025 + 1.75 = 2$

CASE STUDY

CASE 3
Calculate the following percentages.

QUESTION 1. What is 20% of 76?

QUESTION 2. What percent is 98 of 201?

QUESTION 3. What is 44% of 104?

QUESTION 4. What percent is 35 of 79?

QUESTION 5. What percent is 21 of 178?

QUESTION 6. What is 23% of 152?

QUESTION 7. What is 49% of 24?

QUESTION 8. What percent is 231 of 254?

QUESTION 9. What is 76% of 524?

QUESTION 10. What percent is 152 of 324?

ANSWERS

1. 15.2

2. 49%

3. 45.76

4. 44%

5. 12%

6. 34.96

7. 11.76

8. 91%

9. 398.24

10. 47%

FINAL CHECK-UP

1. The health care facility ordered two pizzas for patients. Each pizza has eight slices if four patients each ate three slices. What fraction of the two pizzas was eaten by these patients?

    A. 12/16
    B. 2/5
    C. 1/8
    D. 4/16

2. Dietary delivered a cake that is to be shared between the staff and the patients. Only one staff member wanted a piece of cake, which was 1/12 of the cake. The rest of the patients ate 7/12 of the cake. What fraction of the cake remained?

    A. 7/8
    B. 6/12
    C. 3/12
    D. 4/12

3. The patients ate a tray of baked ziti and had ½ the tray left over. The next day the patients ate 1/3 of what was left. The patients ate the remaining baked ziti on the third day. How much baked ziti did patients eat on the third day?

    A. 1/5
    B. 1/6
    C. 1/4
    D. 1/3

4. There are 24 patients on the unit. On the average 0.5 patients ask for 6 oz of orange juice in the morning. How many 6 oz containers of orange juice should you order?

    A. 12 containers
    B. 60 containers
    C. 24 containers
    D. 12.5 containers

5. Dietary delivered six green plates, three blue plates, three yellow plates, and four white plates. What fraction of plates are not white plates?

    A. 10/16
    B. 11/16
    C. 12/16
    D. 3/5

6. A patient weighs 108 lb. The practitioner orders a diet that will increase the patient's weight by 1.4 during the patient's stay in the hospital. What is the patient's weight goal?

A. 110.5 lb
B. 110 lb
C. 151.2 lb
D. 151.5 lb

7. There are 24 patients on the unit. Hypertension was diagnosed to 7 patients. Diabetes was diagnosed to 15 patients. The rest of the patients were diagnosed with obesity. What fraction of the patients was diagnosed with obesity?

A. 12/24
B. 1/24
C. 3/24
D. 2/24

8. Dietary delivers a bag of plastic utensils. 1/10 of the bag is yellow and 1/5 of the bag is white. What fraction of all the plastic utensils are yellow and white?

A. 5/10
B. 2/10
C. 3/10
D. 2/5

9. About how many patients can be administered medication by the nurse in an hour if it takes the nurse 8.3 minutes to administer medication to one patient?

A. 6.5 patients
B. 7 patients
C. 9 patients
D. 6.8 patients

10. The nurse manager was told by administration to expect a 30% increase in patients on her unit. The unit has an average census of 24 patients. How many more patients should the manager expect to receive?

A. Approximately four more patients
B. Approximately seven more patients
C. Approximately nine more patients
D. Approximately five more patients

CORRECT ANSWERS AND RATIONALES

1. A. 12/16; Hint: Combine the slices of both pizzas (16 slices)
2. D. 4/12; Hint: Subtraction
3. B. 1/6; Hint: Multiplication
4. A. 12 containers; Hint: 24 patients × 0.5 patients
5. C. 12/16; Hint: Add together all plates (16 plates), then add together plates that are not white (12).
6. C. 151.2 lb; Hint: 108 lb × 1.4
7. D. 2/24; Hint: Add the numerators 7 and 15 (22/24), then subtract 22/24 from 24/24.
8. C. 3/10; Hint: Find the common denominator (10), then add the numerators (1/10 and 2/10).
9. B. 7 patients; Hint 60 minutes ÷ 8.3 minutes
10. B. Approximately seven more patients; Hint 24 patients × 0.3 = 7.2 patients

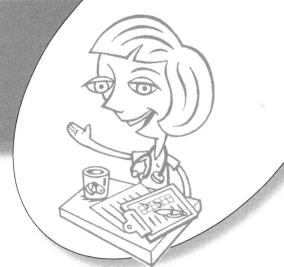

chapter 12

Ratios and Proportions

> ## KEY TERMS
>
> Calculating Proportions   Writing Ratios
> Decreasing Proportions

1. Understanding Ratios

A ratio defines the comparison of two things. Nurse-to-patient ratio is a common ratio used by administrators in a health care facility to describe the number of nurses required to care for a specific number of patients.

A ratio is a mathematical expression for a written statement that compares two things. The expression defines how these things are compared to each other. The comparisons commonly written in a health care facility are the number of nurses to care for a specific number of patients.

A ratio can be used to describe a standard such as a nurse-to-patient ratio of 1:8. A ratio can also be used to describe an empirical relationship between two things. Empirical means describing reality. For example, the ratio between nurse to patient on the West Wing unit during the 7 AM shift today is 1:12.

Writing Ratios

It is common to speak of a relationship between two things by using "to" such as a nurse-to-patient relationship. There are three components to this statement. These are the first thing, "to", and the second thing. Things in the example are nurse and patient.

A ratio also has three elements. These are the first thing, a colon, and the second thing. Notice that the ratio is very similar to the written statement except "to" is replaced with a colon as shown here:

Nurse To Patient

Nurse: Patient

The order of elements in a ratio is critical to the comparison of two things. Let's say our written statement describes one nurse to eight patients relationship. This is written as 1:8. Suppose these are transposed in the ratio such as 8:1. The person reading the ratio expects the ratio to describe the nurse-to-patient relationship. Therefore, this ratio is saying there are eight nurses to one patient.

> **NURSING ALERT**
>
> A ratio can also be written as a fraction such as 1/8 instead of 1:8. It is better to write a ratio as 1:8 when defining a relationship between two things. You write a ratio as a fraction when performing a calculation using proportions.

2. Proportions and Ratios

In the real world, certain relationships between two things produce a desired outcome. For example, one nurse can care for eight patients during a shift based on empirical data. That is, the manager tried different ratios and measured the outcome of each. The most desirable patient care occurred when one nurse cared for eight patients. Therefore, 1:8 ratio between nurse and patients is used as a standard for the manager when staffing the unit.

The 1:8 nurse-to-patients ratio can be restated as saying that the nurse-to-patient ratio is proportional based on the manager's staffing standard. Now suppose there are 16 patients on the unit for the next shift. If staffing doesn't change, then the new ratio will be 1:16 otherwise stated as 1 nurse to 16 patients. This is disproportional to the staffing ratio of 1:8.

The manager must make the staffing to patient ratio for the next shift proportional to the standard staffing ratio. The manager does this by using proportions.

Calculating Proportions

Think of proportions as a recipe for making a cake. A cake has ingredients the amount of each is clearly defined in the recipe. The relationships of ingredients are specified as a ratio. If you want to make a 12 in cake, then use the ratio of ingredients specified in the recipe. But what if you want to make an 18 in cake? You need to proportionally increase the amount of ingredients based on the ratio of ingredients.

Let's see how this is done using the nurse-to-patient ratio. The question is, how many nurses are needed to care for 16 patients? Write the question as fractions rather than ratio as shown in Figure 12–1. You can also write the proportion expression as:

$$x:16 = 1:8$$

$$\frac{X \text{ nurse}}{16 \text{ patients}} = \frac{1 \text{ nurse}}{8 \text{ patients}}$$

$$X \text{ nurse} = \frac{\overset{2}{\cancel{16}} \text{ patients}}{1} \times \frac{1 \text{ nurse}}{\underset{1}{\cancel{8}} \text{ patients}} = 2 \text{ nurses}$$

$$\frac{2 \text{ nurses}}{16 \text{ patients}} = 2 \text{ nurses} : 16 \text{ patients}$$

FIGURE 12–1 • Using the standard ratio of nurse to patient, you can use proportion to calculate the number of nurses required to care for 16 patients.

Here are the steps to find the number of nurses required to care for 16 patients.

1. 1/8 is the same as 1:8 (one nurse to eight patients).
2. Write the target ratio as a fraction. Use x as a place holder for the unknown number of nurses.
3. Solve for the unknown number of nurses (solve for x).
4. Denominator in the fraction is 16 patients. Remember that a fraction is another way to express division. That is, x divided by 16. This is important to remember because you reverse the arithmetic when moving a number to the opposite side of the equal sign.
5. Move the 16 to the right of the equal sign and reverse the operation from division to multiplication.
6. Divide 8 patients into 16 patients. The result is 2.
7. Multiple the number of nurses (1) by 2. The result is 2 nurses. Therefore, x is equal to 2.
8. Rewrite the new ratio replacing x with 2. The number of nurses needed to care for 16 patients are 2 nurses.

NURSING ALERT

The assumption is that as long as the relationship between two things remains the same (proportional), then the outcome should be the same. That is, 2 nurses should deliver the same level of care for 16 patients as the level of care 1 nurse gives to 8 patients. Sometimes, this is not true. Although the relationship is the same based on the ratio, other factors may influence the outcome.

Decreasing Proportions

Decreasing proportions is performed when one thing in the relationship decreases in size. Let's say that the West Wing unit has 2 nurses for 16 patients. Patients discharged were 8 and now there are 8 patients. How many nurses are required to care for 8 patients if the nurse-to-patient relationship remains proportional? Also assume you don't know the standard nurse-to-patient ratio.

To determine the number of nurses you'll need, you assume that the relationship between nurse to patient remains proportional to the 2 nurse to 16 patient ratio that exists on this shift.

Write the problem as shown in Figure 12–2. This is very similar to the previous example except you are decreasing the number of nurses required for the shift.

Here are the steps to find the number of nurses required to care for 8 patients.

1. 2/16 is the same as 2:16 (2 nurses to 16 patients).

2. Write the target ratio as a fraction. Use x as a place holder for the unknown number of nurses.

3. Solve for the unknown number of nurses (solve for x).

4. The denominator in the fraction is 8 patients. Remember that a fraction is another way to express division. That is, x divided by 8. This is important to remember because you reverse the arithmetic when moving a number to the opposite side of the equal sign.

5. Move 8 to the right of the equal sign and reverse the operation from division to multiplication.

$$\frac{X \text{ nurse}}{8 \text{ patients}} = \frac{2 \text{ nurses}}{16 \text{ patients}}$$

$$X \text{ nurse} = \frac{\overset{1}{\cancel{8}} \text{ patients}}{1} \times \frac{2 \text{ nurses}}{\underset{2}{\cancel{16}} \text{ patients}} = 1 \text{ nurse}$$

$$\frac{1 \text{ nurse}}{8 \text{ patients}} = 1 \text{ nurse} : 8 \text{ patients}$$

FIGURE 12–2 • Calculate the answer by moving the 8 to the right and reversing the operation.

6. Divide 8 patients into 8, which result in 1 and divide 8 into 16 patients. The result is 2.

7. Divide 2 nurses by 2 patients. The result is 1 nurse. Therefore, x is equal to 1.

8. Rewrite the new ratio replacing x with 1. The number of nurses need to care for 8 patients is 1 nurse.

CASE STUDY

CASE 1
Calculate the following proportions.

QUESTION 1. x:8 = 2:4; x =

QUESTION 2. x:24 = 2:16; x =

QUESTION 3. x:20 = 22:40; x =

QUESTION 4. x:15 = 3:5; x =

QUESTION 5. x:36 = 1:9; x =

QUESTION 6. x:20 = 1:5; x =

QUESTION 7. x:64 = 1:32; x =

QUESTION 8. 3:x = 1:6; x =

QUESTION 9. x:7 = 3:14; x =

QUESTION 10. x:18 = 22:36; x =

ANSWERS

1. x:8 = 2:4; x = 4

2. x:24 = 2:16; x = 3

3. x:20 = 22:40; x = 11

4. x:15 = 3:5; x = 9

5. x:36 = 1:9; x = 4

6. x:20 = 1:5; x = 4

7. x:64 = 1:32; x = 2

8. 3:x = 1:6; x = 18

9. x:7 = 3:14; x = 1.5

10. x:18 = 22:36; x = 11

FINAL CHECK-UP

1. The dietician uses the ratio of 2 hamburgers:patient. Your unit has 18 patients. How many hamburgers do you expect to receive?

   A. 26 hamburgers
   B. 36 hamburgers
   C. 46 hamburgers
   D. 16 hamburgers

2. The health care facility has a ratio of 1 CNA:2 Nurses and a ratio of 1 nurse: 8 patients. Your unit has 16 patients. How many CNAs would you schedule?

   A. 4 CNAs
   B. 3 CNAs
   C. 2 CNAs
   D. 1 CNA

3. A bag of normal saline contains 1000 L. The practitioner order 200 L/hr. How many hours will it take to infuse 1000 L?

   A. 5 hours
   B. 6 hours
   C. 12 hours
   D. 4 hours

4. The emergency department has two practitioners per shift. On the average the department sees 30 patients per hour. What is the ratio of patients to practitioners?

   A. 2:30
   B. 30:2
   C. 1:30
   D. 30:1

5. The health care facility has 1 nurse manager for every 48 patients. The health care facility also has a ratio of 1 nurse to 8 patients. What is the ratio of nurse manager to nurses?

   A. 1 nurse manager:12 nurses

   B. 1 nurse manager:4 nurses

   C. 1 nurse manager:8 nurses

   D. 1 nurse manager:6 nurses

6. Problem 4 states that the emergency department has two practitioners per shift. On the average, the department sees 30 patients per hour. The nurse manager of the emergency department receives word of a massive traffic accident and to expect 150 patients. How many practitioners are needed to staff the emergency department for the next hour?

   A. 12 practitioners

   B. 6 practitioners

   C. 24 practitioners

   D. 8 practitioners

7. The practitioner order 650 mg of acetaminophen. The pharmacy sends 1 tablet of 352 mg of acetaminophen. How many tablets do you need to administer to the patient?

   A. 2 tablets

   B. 1.5 tablets

   C. 2.5 tablets

   D. 1 tablet

8. During the day shift, the health care facility has 30 respiratory therapists on duty. There are also 240 patients. What is the ratio of one therapist to patient?

   A. 10 patients

   B. 18 patients

   C. 12 patients

   D. 8 patients

9. A nurse can administer 20 tablets of medication to one patient in 15 minutes. The nurse is assigned 12 patients all receiving approximately the same number of medications. How long will it take the nurse to administer medication to all his patients?

   A. 92 minutes

   B. 90 minutes

   C. 108 minutes

   D. 180 minutes

10. **The West Wing unit has 64 patients. An emergency situation required the manager to reassign two nurses from the West Wing unit. The standard nurse-to-patient ratio is 1:8. What is the approximate nurse-to-patient ratio on the West Wing unit after nurses are reassigned?**

    A. 1 nurse:6 patients
    B. 1 nurse:11 patients
    C. 1 nurse:12 patients
    D. 1 nurse:16 patients

CORRECT ANSWERS AND RATIONALES

   1. B. 36 hamburgers; Hint: x:18 patients = 2 hamburgers:1 patient
   2. D. 1 CNA; Hint: x:16 patients = 0.5 CNA:8 patients
   3. A. 5 hours; Hint: 1000 L:x = 200 L:1 hour
   4. B. 30:2; Hint: Patients to practitioners
   5. D. 1 nurse manager:6 nurses; Hint: x:48 patients = 1 nurse:8 patients
   6. A. 12 practitioners; Hint: x:150 patients = 2 practitioners:30 patients
   7. A. 2 tablets; Hint: x:650 mg = 1 tablet:325 mg
   8. D. 8 patients; Hint: 240 patients ÷ 30 respiratory therapists = 8 patients
   9. D. 180 minutes; Hint: x:12 patients = 15 minutes:1 patient
  10. B. 1 nurse:11 patients; Hint: There were originally 8 nurses to 64 patients, which is 1 nurse:8 patients. Now there are 6 nurses to 64 patients. 64 patients ÷ 6 nurses = 10.7 patients or approximately 1 nurse to 11 patients.

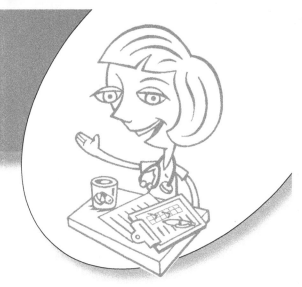

chapter 13

Equations

LEARNING OBJECTIVES

1. Understanding Equations
2. Algebraic Expression
3. Identifying the Unknown
4. Order of Operations

> ### KEY TERMS
>
> Algebraic Equation   Operators
> Algebraic Equation and Variables   Parentheses
> Finding the Unknown   Variables

1. Understanding Equations

An **equation** is an expression of equality using numbers, symbols, and mathematical operations. At first the concept of an equation may seem challenging to understand; however, let's explore this concept in plain English.

You can say that: Bob is the same age as Mary. This is an equation because you are saying that Bob and Mary are of the same age. You can write this as a mathematical equation as: Bob's age = Mary's age. In this example, the equal sign (=) is referred to as the equivalent operator. Values on both the left side and the right side of the equal sign are the same.

Notice that words are used in place of numbers in the equation Bob's age = Mary's age. Typically, values are used in place of words such as 23 = 23 but this wouldn't communicate much because no one would know the meaning of the values 23.

A more common equation expresses a mathematical operation such as:

$$2 + 20 = 23$$

Operators

An **operator** is a mathematical symbol that tells the reader to perform an operation such as addition (+) or a comparison such as the equivalent operator (=) using values in the equation. Values are referred to as operands. An **operand** is something the operator is affecting. Bob's age and Mary's age are operands. The equivalent operator is an operator saying that the left side value is equal to the right side value. Collectively operands and operators form an equation.

Both the English sentence and the equation say the same things.

English: Bob is the same age as Mary.
Equation: Bob's age = Mary's age

An equation is a statement of equality because an equation compares two things—Bob's age and Mary's age. The equivalent operator (equals sign) is used if both values (operands) are the same. However, there are times when the values are different. The equation is still used to compare values except the operator is different based on the difference in the values.

If the operand on the left (Bob's age) is higher than the operand on the right (Mary's age), then the greater than (>) operator is used. Here's how the equation is written:

English: Bob's age is greater than Mary's age.
Equation: Bob's age > Mary's age

If the operand on the left (Bob's age) is lower than the operand on the right (Mary's age), then the less than (<) operation is used. Here's how the equation is written:

English: Bob's age is less than Mary's age.
Equation: Bob's age < Mary's age

Table 13–1 contains common operators used in equations.

Variables

The equation $2 + 20 = 23$ contains all the elements of the equation. That is, there is nothing more to do with the equation because all elements are known. Many equations have most but not all elements requiring you to calculate the missing element—calculate the unknown value.

Let's say you are asked to calculate Bob's age. The problem states that Bob is 2 years younger than Mary. Mary is 23 years old. You can write the equation as

$$23 \text{ years} - 2 \text{ years} = x$$

TABLE 13–1 Here is a List of Common Operators Used in Common Equations	
Operators	Operations
+	Addition
−	Subtraction
× or *	Multiplication
/	Division
!=	Not equal to
<	Less than
>	Greater than
<=	Less than or equal to
>=	Greater than or equal to

A variable is used as a placeholder for the unknown value in the equation. A **variable** is a symbol, which is usually a letter that takes the place of an unknown number in an equation. In this example, the letter x is used as the placeholder for Bob's age.

A variable can change value in an equation. A number is a constant. A **constant** is part of an equation that cannot change. For example, 23 is a number that will always have one value, which is 23. The variable x can have a different value each time the x is used in the equation.

You are usually asked to "solve for x." This means that you need to perform the operations specified in equation to determine the value of the variable. In this example, you subtract 2 from Mary's age of 23 years to arrive at Bob's age, which is 21 years. You can then say that

$$\text{Bob's age} = x = 21 \text{ years}$$

NURSING ALERT

Any letter can be used to represent the variable. Some equations may have more than one unknown. Each unknown must be represented by a unique letter.

---

2. Algebraic Expression

An **expression** is a mathematical statement that shows a relationship between two or more values. An **algebraic expression** is an expression that uses letters (variables) to represent numbers and operators. Let's return to Bob and Mary to see how to create an algebraic expression.

In an English statement, you say that Bob is the same age as Mary. You can write this English statement as an algebraic expression by using letters (variables) to represent Bob's age and Mary's age.

First, define each variable such as:

$$a = \text{Bob's age}$$
$$b = \text{Mary's age}$$

Next, create the algebraic expression using the letters in place of Bob's age and Mary's age such as:

$$a = b$$

Someone reading a = b will be in doubt or be confused about the meaning of the algebraic expression unless the person knows the definitions of a and b.

Once the definitions are known the person realizes that the algebraic expression means:

$$\text{Bob's age} = \text{Mary's age}$$

The use of letters in an algebraic expression is arguably the most difficult aspect of algebraic expressions to understand because at first reading the algebraic expression seems meaningless. That is, until you know the definitions of each letter.

Take the following algebraic expression as an example:

$$wl = A$$

You might feel intimated if someone wrote that algebraic expression on the board and then began talking about its meaning as if you understood this algebraic expression. As you're trying to make sense of the letters, the speaker is talking about how to apply the algebraic expression in real life situations.

Now let's translate the algebraic expression into an English statement by first defining each letter.

$$w = \text{width}$$
$$l = \text{length}$$
$$A = \text{area}$$

Next, write the algebraic expression as an English statement:
Width multiply length is equal to the area.

The algebraic expression in the following example shows the relationship between width, length, and area:

$$wl = A$$

NURSING ALERT

Placing two letters (variables) next to each other in an algebraic expression implies that the values represented by the letters are multiplied. Here wl means multiply width by length.

An algebraic expression is sometimes referred to as a formula. A **formula** describes relationships among values. The algebraic expression $wl = A$ is a formula for calculating the area of a rectangle.

Algebraic Equation

You'll recall that an expression is a mathematical statement that shows a relationship between two or more values. An expression cannot be solved.

An algebraic equation is similar to an algebraic expression except the algebraic equation can be solved.

For example, the algebraic expression wl = A shows the relationship between width, length, and area. The algebraic expression is considered an algebraic equation when values are used as shown here because you can solve the equation:

$$5 \text{ ft} \times 10 \text{ ft} = A$$
$$A = 50 \text{ sq ft}$$

Algebraic Equation and Variables

An algebraic equation uses variables instead of actual values. Each variable is represented by a letter that is assigned a value. The letter is then used in the algebraic equation as a placeholder for the value.

Let's rewrite the algebraic equation for the area of a rectangle using variables instead of values. Notice that a variable is defined before the variable is used in the algebraic equation.

$$w = 5 \text{ ft}$$
$$l = 10 \text{ ft}$$
$$w \times l = A$$

Each variable is replaced by the corresponding value in the algebraic equation before solving the algebraic equation.

> **NURSING ALERT**
>
> Any letter can be used to represent a variable; however, it is best to use a letter that relates to the value represented by the variable. For example, you could use the letters "y" and "z" to represent width and length in the algebraic equation but "w" and "l" are better choices because each gives a hint as to what the value represents (width and length).

3. Identifying the Unknown

There is at least one unknown value in algebraic equation, which is usually identified as a variable (letter) in the equation. You are probably familiar with the unknown value being written to the right of the equal sign such as in the following equation:

$$5 \text{ ft} \times 10 \text{ ft} = A$$

However, the unknown value can be written elsewhere in the algebraic equation. Part of the operation to solve the equation is to rewrite the equation so that the unknown is by itself on one side or the other side of equal sign.

The position of the unknown in the algebraic equation is related to the corresponding algebraic expression. Let's revisit the following algebraic expression. This algebraic expression shows the relationship between width, length, and area of a rectangle.

$$wl = A$$

Let's translate this algebraic expression to an algebraic equation. The known values are the length of 10 ft and the area of 50 sq ft. The unknown value is the width. Insert values into the algebraic expression. Notice that the variable identified by the letter w is within the equation and not positioned by itself either left or right of the equal sign. This is fine for now until you begin to solve the equation.

$$w \times 10 \text{ ft} = 50 \text{ sq ft}$$

Finding the Unknown

An algebraic equation usually has one unknown value, although there can be multiple unknown values in complex algebraic equations. Complex algebraic equations are beyond the scope of this book.

Before attempting to solve the equation, you need to have the unknown value by itself on one side of the equal sign. In the following equation, you need to move 10 ft to the right side of the equal sign so that the "w" is by itself on the left side of the equal sign.

$$w \times 10 \text{ ft} = 50 \text{ sq ft}$$

You move values to the other side of the equal sign by performing the opposite operation to both sides of the equation. Understandably this sounds confusing but it really isn't.

The operation in the equation is multiplication. That is, $w \times 10$ ft is the operation. The opposite operation is division. That is, each site of the equation must be divided by 10.

On the left side of the equal sign, divide 10 ft by 10, which result in 0. The left side of the equation is now:

$$w = 50 \text{ sq ft}$$

Next, divide the value on the right side of the equal sign by 10. That is, 50 sq ft/10, which results in 5. The equation is now:

$$w = 5 \text{ ft}$$

The unknown value of "w" is 5 ft.

The same process can be used to find the unknown value using other operations such as division, addition, and subtraction.

4. Order of Operations

An equation can have multiple operations within the equation such as in this next example. Solving the equation seems straightforward since the equation contains all the values and the unknown value "x" is by itself on the right side of the equal sign.

$$8 + 5 \times 6 = x$$

But is this equation as straightforward as it seems? What is the value of x? Is it 38? Is it 78? Either answer might be correct depending on the order in which the calculations are performed.

$$8 + 5 = 13 \text{ and } 13 \times 6 = 78$$
$$5 \times 6 = 30 \text{ and } 30 + 8 = 38$$

The answer is different depending on which calculation is performed first. The order in which calculations are performed in an equation is determined by the order of operations. The order of operations is a rule that defines when each calculation is performed.

Let's apply the order of operations to this equation to calculate the value of "x."

$$8 + 5 \times 6 = x$$

First, there are no parentheses in the equation; therefore, the first order of operations can be ignored.

Order	Operation
TABLE 13–2	The Order of Operations Determines When Each Calculation is Performed in an Equation
1	Perform calculations that are within parentheses. If there are parentheses within parentheses (nested parentheses), then calculate the innermost parentheses and work your way to the outermost parentheses.
2	Perform multiplication and division working from left to right.
3	Perform addition and subtraction working from left to right.

Next, perform multiplication.

$$5 \times 6 = 30$$

And then perform addition.

$$30 + 8 = 38$$
$$x = 38$$

Notice how the order of operations takes the guesswork out of solving an equation.

Parentheses

You can clarify the order that you want calculations performed in an equation by placing calculations within parentheses. Based on the order of operations, calculations within parentheses are performed before calculations that are outside parentheses.

Let's see how to use parentheses in this expression. You already know that multiplication is performed before addition according to the order of operations. However, suppose you want the addition to be performed first. You can make this happen by placing the addition calculation within parentheses such as:

$$(8 + 5) \times 6 = x$$

Now this equation is calculated as:

$$8 + 5 = 13$$
$$13 \times 6 = 78$$
$$x = 78$$

An equation can have multiple sets of parentheses each further clarifying the desired order of calculations. It is a good practice to keep the result of the calculation within the parentheses while solving the equation as illustrated in the next equation.

$$(8 + 5) \times (6 + 4) = x$$

From left to right perform the calculations within the parenthesis first.

$$(13) \times (6 + 4) = x$$
$$(13) \times (10) = x$$

Notice that the parentheses remain after performing the calculation within the parentheses. This helps to clarify the remaining calculation in the equation. You can then remove the parentheses and perform the multiplication.

$$13 \times 10 = 130$$
$$x = 130$$

CASE STUDY

CASE 1

Calculate the following equations.

QUESTION 1. $56 + 20 \times (2 + 32) =$

QUESTION 2. $x + 4 = 8$

QUESTION 3. $(3 \times 5) + (6 - 2) \times 2 =$

QUESTION 4. $y \times 8 = 16$

QUESTION 5. $25 + z = 125$

QUESTION 6. $(75 - 23)/(4) =$

QUESTION 7. $82 - x = (5 + 10)$

QUESTION 8. $(3 \times 24) + d = 72$

QUESTION 9. $15 \times (2 + 5) =$

QUESTION 10. $18/2 + (45 + 5) =$

ANSWERS

1. $56 + 20 \times (2 + 32) =$
    $56 + 20 \times (4) =$
    $56 + 80 = 136$

2. $x + 4 = 8$
    $x = 8 - 4$
    $x = 4$

3. $(3 \times 5) + (6 - 2) \times 2 =$
   $(15) + (4) \times 2 =$
   $15 + 8 = 23$

4. $y \times 8 = 16$
   $y = 16/8$
   $y = 2$

5. $25 + z = 125$
   $z = 125 - 25$
   $z = 100$

6. $(75 - 23)/(4) =$
   $52/4 = 13$

7. $82 - x = (5 + 10)$
   $82 - x = (15)$
   $x = 15 + 82$
   $x = 97$

8. $(3 \times 24) + d = 72$
   $(72) + d = 72$
   $d = 72 - 72$
   $d = 0$

9. $15 \times (2 + 5) =$
   $15 \times (7) = 105$

10. $18/2 + (45 + 5) =$
    $18/2 + (50) =$
    $9 + 50 = 59$

FINAL CHECK-UP

1. The health care facility developed a formula for determining CNA staffing levels. The expression is used to describe the relationships among the number of patients, CNA assignment, and required number of CNAs. How many CNAs are required for 20 patients and a CNA assignment of 0.1?

   Number of Patients X CNA Assignment = Required Number of CNAs

   A. 2 CNAs
   B. 4 CNAs
   C. 5 CNAs
   D. 6 CNAs

2. **Refer to the expression in problem 1. If the nurse manager scheduled 5 CNAs, how many patients are on the unit?**

    A. 32 patients

    B. 30 patients

    C. 25 patients

    D. 50 patients

3. **There are 98 patients. The nurse manager uses 1 nurse to 8 patient ratio and 1 CNA to 12 patients. Write an expression that shows the relationship between patients, nurses, CNAs, and the total number of clinical staff (nurse and CNAs) required to care for patients?**

    A. $98 \times 8 \times 12 =$ Total Number of Clinical Staff

    B. (Number of Patients/8) + (Number of Patients/12) = Total Number of Clinical Staff

    C. $98 + 8 + 12 =$ Total Number of Clinical Staff

    D. (Number of Patients $\times$ 8) $\times$ (Number of Patients $\times$ 12) = Total Number of Clinical Staff

4. **Using the expression you created in problem 3, calculate the number of nurses and CNAs required to care for 96 patients.**

    A. 24 total number of clinical staff

    B. 10 total number of clinical staff

    C. 20 total number of clinical staff

    D. 24.5 total number of clinical staff

5. **The nurse manager wrote the following equation but forgot to label values in the equation. You are told to calculate the equation to determine the number of juice boxes that are expected to be delivered by dietary. How many boxes of juice will be delivered? $8 \times 5 + 3 =$ Total boxes of juice**

    A. 64

    B. 43

    C. 55

    D. 66

6. **Write an expression that shows the following relationship. Total time needed to administer medication for all patients on the day shift is the sum of the time spent on each medication pass. The nurse spends 20 minutes per patient administering morning meds; 10 minutes per patient administering noon meds; 5 minutes per patient administering 2 PM medications; and 2 minutes per patient during the shift administering PRN medication.**

    A. (Number of Patients/20 min) + (Number of Patients/10 min) + (Number of Patients/5 min) + (Number of Patients/2 min) = Total Time to Administer Medication to All Patients on the Day Shift

    B. (Number of Patients + 20 min) $\times$ (Number of Patients + 10 min) $\times$ (Number of Patients + 5 min) $\times$ (Number of Patients + 2 min) = Total Time to Administer Medication to All Patients on the Day shift

C. (Number of Patients + 20 min) + (Number of Patients + 10 min) + (Number of Patients + 5 min) + (Number of Patients + 2 min) = Total Time to Administer Medication to All Patients on the Day shift

D. (Number of Patients × 20 min) + (Number of Patients × 10 min) + (Number of Patients × 5 min) + (Number of Patients × 2 min) = Total Time to Administer Medication to All Patients on the Day Shift

7. **Staffing requirements for nurses is based on the acuity of the patient. The acuity is assessed by the patient's diagnosis, which reflects the amount of time the nurse will likely spend per shift caring for the patient. For an average patient the acuity factor is 1. For an unstable patient the acuity factor is 2 and for a critically ill patient the acuity factor is 4. The acuity factor is divided into the normal eight patient assignment per nurse to determine the number of patients per nurse is assigned. Write the expression that shows the relationship between the number of critically ill patients that will be assigned to a nurse.**

   A. 4/8 = number of patients per nurse
   B. 8/4 = number of patients per nurse
   C. 2/8 = number of patients per nurse
   D. 8/2 = number of patients per nurse

8. **Based on problem 7, write an equation that determines the number of nurses required to care for 16 average patients; 12 unstable patients; and 4 critically ill patients.**

   A. (16 + (8/1)) + (12 + (8/2)) + (4 + (8/4)) = Total Number of Nurses
   B. (16/(8/1)) + (12/(8/2)) + (4/(8/4)) = Total Number of Nurses
   C. (16 + (8/1)) × (12 + (8/2)) × (4 + (8/4)) = Total Number of Nurses
   D. (16 × (8/1)) × (12 × (8/2)) × (4 × (8/4)) = Total Number of Nurses

9. **Refer to problem 8. What is the total number of nurses required to care for those patients?**

   A. 7 nurses
   B. 5 nurses
   C. 9 nurses
   D. 8 nurses

10. **Refer to Problem 6. If there were 30 patients on the unit, calculate the length of the time spent administering medications on the day shift.**

    A. 1100 minutes
    B. 1111 minutes
    C. 1010 minutes
    D. 1110 minutes

CORRECT ANSWERS AND RATIONALES

1. A. 2 CNAs; Hint: $20 \times 0.1 = 2$ CNAs

2. D. 50 patients; Hint: $x \times 0.1 = 5$ CNAs, then $x = 5/0.1$

3. B. (Number of Patients/8) + (Number of Patients/12) = Total Number of Clinical Staff; Hint: An expression shows a relationship.

4. C. 20 total number of clinical staff; Hint: (96 patients/8) + (96 patients/12) = Total Number of Clinical Staff, then (12 nurses) + (8 CNAs) = 20 total number of clinical staff

5. B. 43; Hint: Order of operations

6. D. (Number of Patients × 20 min) + (Number of Patients × 10 min) + (Number of Patients × 5 min) + (Number of Patients × 2 min) = Total Time to Administer Medication to All Patients on the Day Shift

7. B. (8/4) = number of patients per nurse; Hint: 8 patients' normal assignments divided by the acuity factor of 4.

8. B. (16/(8/1)) + (12/(8/2)) + (4/(8/4)) = Total Number of Nurses; Hint: Calculations in the innermost parentheses are calculated first, then perform the calculations in the outer parentheses.

9. A. 7 nurses

   (16/(8/1)) + (12/(8/2)) + (4/(8/4)) = Total Number of Nurses

   (16/(8)) + (12/(4)) + (4/(2)) = Total Number of Nurses

   (2 nurses) + (3 nurses) + (2 nurses) = 7 Nurses

10. A. 1110 minutes; Hint: (30 × 20 min) + (30 × 10 min) + (30 × 5 min) + (30 × 2 min) = Total Time to Administer Medication to All Patients on the Day Shift

    (600 min) + (300 min) + (150 min) + (60 min) = Total Time to Administer Medication to All Patients on the Day Shift

    1110 minutes = 18.5 hours = Total Time to Administer Medication to All Patients on the Day Shift

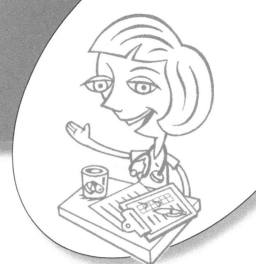

Answering Tricky Questions

All dose calculation questions that you'll be asked on a test can be solved using formulas learned in this book or by using basic math that you learned in grammar school. However, some questions are purposely written to confuse you. Unfair!

Maybe, but the goal is to test your critical thinking skills because in the real world dose calculation problems aren't always presented to you in a clear, concise format. Instead you might be given a bunch of values and you have to pick out those values that are needed to calculate your patient's dose.

In this chapter, you'll see tricky questions that are similar to those that you find on tests and you'll learn ways of solving those questions.

1. Too Many Numbers

You are bound to encounter a question that is purposely designed to confuse you by providing more information than you need to answer the question. The challenge is to select the correct formula and values from the clutter of information in the question.

Here's an example:

Your patient's serum potassium level has been declining. The latest lab shows a serum potassium level of 3.5. Although this is at the low end of the normal range, the physician writes an order for 30 mEq of potassium chloride to be added to 1000 mL of normal saline and administered to your patient over 12 hours. The pharmacy delivers 40 mEq of potassium chloride per 20 mL. How many milliliters of potassium chloride will you administer to your patient?

Probably the first two pieces of information that pop out are 1000 mL and 12 hours. Isn't there a formula that requires converting hours to minutes then divide minutes into milliliters?

Sure there is. But is that the formula needed to answer this question? No. The formula that uses these values calculates the pump setting, which is not what you are asked to calculate. These values are distracters designed to stress you. The information looks like it should be used in the calculation, but you're not sure how to use it—and that's because the information doesn't help you answer the question.

The next two pieces of information that grab your attention are 30 mEq and 1000 mL. Do you divide 30 mEq into 1000 mL? Unsure? This too is a distraction designed to mislead you from the values you really need for the calculation. Why would you divide 30 mEq into 1000 mL? If you can't answer this question, then you are probably on the wrong track.

The question is how many milliliters of potassium chloride will you administer to your patient? The pharmacy delivers 40 mEq of potassium chloride per 20 mL. This is what you have on hand, so you know this must be a component of your calculation. If so, then what did the physician order? 30 mEq potassium chloride. You picked out from the problem the amount ordered and the amount on hand. A bell should sound in your head reminding you of a formula that uses these values.

$$15 \text{ mL} = \frac{30 \text{ mEq}}{40 \text{ mEq}} \times 20 \text{ mL}$$

2. The Sleight of Hand

Another type of question that you must be prepared to handle is a question whose solution doesn't seem to fit any of the formulas that you are learned. It leaves you scratching your head saying, why should they ask such a dumb question. Whether the question is dumb or not, you must calculate the results that the question poses.

Here's an example:

How many hours does it take for 2 L of normal saline to infuse if the physician writes an order to infuse 2000 mL of normal saline at 125 mL/hr?

At first glance you may say, who cares? If the physician set the amount (1000 mL) and rate (125 mL per hour), then simply set the pump to 125 mL. This is correct if the question was asking you for the pump setting, but it isn't. Knowing the amount of time the drug is infusing helps the nurse in many ways including scheduling activities with that patient and other patients who are assigned to the nurse.

Again, there are more values in the question then you need to calculate the answer. The clue to answering this question is finding the common value. You are asked how many hours to infuse 2 L. You are told that 125 mL is infused each hour. Both specify time and volume.

There are two pieces of information (stressors) in this question that are designed to confuse you. First is 2000 mL ordered by the physician. This doesn't help you solve the problem. And then there is 2 L of normal saline. If you are rushing to answer this question you might overlook the need to calculate common units of measurement. 2 L refers to 2 liters. The physician's order states mL—milliliters.

Once you convert 2 L to milliliters, you'll quickly notice a similarity to the value ordered by the physician:

$$2000 \text{ mL} = 2 \text{ L} \times 1000$$

You can restate the question:

I have 2000 mL infusing at 125 mL/hr. How many hours will this take?

You won't find a formula in this book or probably any book to solve this problem because the solution requires simple division.

$$16 \text{ hours} = \frac{2000 \text{ mL}}{125 \text{ mL}}$$

NURSING ALERT

If you are asked a question that doesn't seem to be answered by using a dose calculation formula, then think carefully of what you are being asked and then try solving the problem using basic math that you already know.

---

3. The Double Barrel Question

Be alert for a question that asks you two questions in one. You'll be asked to calculate the dose of two different medications that are to be administered to your patient. The objective is to test your critical thinking ability.

Here's the trick to answering the question:

- Identify the two questions that you're being asked to answer.
- Create two columns—one for each drug that you'll be administering according to the question.
- Label the columns with the name of the drug.
- Enter values from the question that pertains to the drug in the corresponding column—be sure to label each value (i.e., ordered and on hand).
- Calculate the dose for each drug—remember that values to calculate the dose of one drug have nothing to do with calculating the dose of the other drug.

4. The Per Dose Question

Some questions are written to test your thinking skills in addition to your ability to calculate the proper dose to administer to your patient. Here's a typical question that you might be asked on a test:

A young patient who weighs 30 lb has an infection and the physician wants you to administer Ampicillin. The physician's order reads Ampicillin 50 mg/kg P.O. per day for 7 days. The pharmacy delivers 100 mg/mL. The daily dose is given every 6 hours. What dose would you administer to your patient every 6 hours?

There is a lot of information in this question, some of which can be misleading unless you read the question carefully. Here are the tricky parts of this question.

The values represent a daily dose—not a single dose you administer to your patient.

You don't divide the daily dose by 6. There are 4 not 6 doses/day.

It is obvious from the question that you use the pediatric formula. Just remember that the result is for the entire day.

$$13.636 \text{ kg} = \frac{30 \text{ lb}}{2.2 \text{ lb}}$$

$$6.818 \text{ mL/day} = \frac{50 \text{ mg} \times 13.636}{100 \text{ mg}} \times 1 \text{ mL}$$

$$1.7 \text{ mL/dose} = \frac{6.818 \text{ mL}}{4 \text{ doses}}$$

HINT: Don't assume that values given in a question pertain to a single dose.

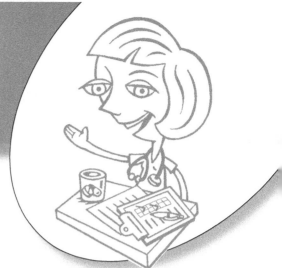

appendix B

Quick Reference

1. Conversion Factors

1 mg = 1000 mcg
1 kg = 2.2 lb
1 g = 60 mg
1/100 g = 0/6 mg
1 in = 2/5 cm
1 cm = 1 mm
1 m = 100 cm
1/150 g = 0/4 mg
1 tsp = 5 mL
1 tbsp = 15 mL
1 oz = 30 mL
1 mm Hg = 1.36 cm H_2O

2. Temperature Conversion Table

Fahrenheit	Celsius
89.6	32
91.4	33
93.2	34
95.0	35
96.8	36
98.6	37
100.4	38
102.2	39
104.2	40
105.8	41

3. Temperature Conversion Formulas

$$\text{Celsius} = (\text{Fahrenheit} - 32) \times 0.5555$$
$$\text{Fahrenheit} = (\text{Celsius} \times 1.8) + 32$$

4. Medication Formulas

Intravenous Drip Rate

$$X \text{ gtt/min} = \frac{\text{volume ordered} \times \text{drip factor}}{\text{minutes to infuse}}$$

Pump Rate

$$\text{Pump rate (mL/hr)} = \frac{\text{volume (mL)}}{\text{time (hr)}}$$

How Much Longer Will the Intravenous Run?

$$\text{Time remaining} = \frac{\text{current volume (mL)}}{\text{pump setting (mL)}}$$

Medication Concentration

$$\text{Concentration} = \frac{\text{drug quantity (g, mg, mcg)}}{\text{volume of solution (mL)}}$$

Dose Calculation

$$\text{Dose} = \frac{\text{ordered}}{\text{on hand}} \times \text{quantity}$$

Weight Based Calculation

$$\text{Dose} = \frac{\text{orders (kg)} \times \text{patient's weight (kg)}}{\text{on hand}} \times \text{quantity on hand}$$

Multi-Dose Formula

$$\text{Dose per day} = \frac{\text{orders (kg)} \times \text{patients's weight (kg)}}{\text{on hand}} \times \text{quantity on hand}$$

$$\text{Dose} = \frac{\text{dose per day}}{\text{ordered number of doses}}$$

Heparin Calculation mL/hr

1. Calculate the number of heparin units in a milliliter.

$$\text{Heparin (U/mL)} = \frac{\text{on hand heparin (U)}}{\text{on hand (mL)}}$$

2. Calculate the number of milliliters to administer per hour.

$$\text{Dose (mL/hr)} = \frac{\text{ordered heparin (U)}}{\text{heparin (U/mL)}}$$

Heparin Calculation in Units

$$\text{Heparin (U/mL)} = \frac{\text{ordered (U)}}{\text{ordered (mL)}}$$

$$\text{Heparin (U)} = \text{heparin (U/mL)} \times \text{ordered (mL/hr)}$$

Heparin Subcutaneous Formula

$$\text{Dose} = \frac{\text{ordered}}{\text{on hand}} \times \text{quantity}$$

Dopamine Formula

1. Convert the patient's weight from pounds to kilograms.

$$\text{Weight (kg)} = \frac{\text{weight (lb)}}{2.2}$$

2. Calculate the concentration of dopamine that is delivered from the pharmacy.

$$\text{Concentration} = \frac{\text{on hand (mg)}}{\text{on hand (mL)}}$$

Body Surface Area Child Dose Calculation Formula

$$\text{Child dose} = \frac{\text{body surface area (m}^2\text{)}}{1.73 \text{ m}^2} \times \text{adult dose}$$

Enteral Food Feeding Dilution Formula

1. Total volume = concentration volume/dilution factor
2. Water to add = total volume − concentration volume

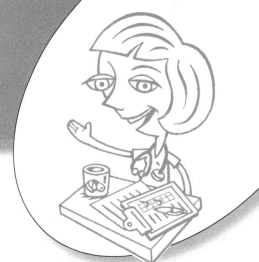

Final Exam Part 1

1. The physician ordered 1000 mL of 0.9% of Sodium Chloride I.V. over 60 mL/hr. On hand is tubing with a 10 gtt/mL drip factor. What drip rate would you use?

2. The physician ordered Quinidine Sulfate 400 mg P.O. daily. The pharmacy delivers Quinidine Sulfate 0.2 g per tablet. How many tablets would you administer to your patient?

3. The physician ordered heparin 5250 U S.C. daily. The medication label reads 15,000 U heparin/5 mL. How many milliliters will you administer to the patient per hour?
   A. 1.25 mL
   B. 1 mL
   C. 1.75 mL
   D. 2 mL

4. The physician ordered Lithostat 120 mg/kg · day q4h. Your patient weighs 110 lb. The pharmacy delivers Lithostat 250 mg/mL. How many milliliters per dose will you administer to your patient?

5. The physician ordered dopamine 7 mcg/kg · min for a patient who weighs 190 lb. The pharmacy delivers dopamine 800 mg in 500 mL D5W. How many milliliters will you administer to your patient per hour?

6. The physician ordered for Vistaril 25 mg and the pharmacy delivered Vistaril 50 mg/mL. What dose would you administer to the patient?

   A. 2 mL

   B. 1.5 mL

   C. 1.0 mL

   D. 0.5 mL

7. The physician ordered 1500 mL normal saline I.V. over 12 hours. What pump setting would you use?

8. The physician ordered Zovirax 10 mg/kg. The patient weighs 77 lb. The medication label reads 100 mg/mL. What dose will you administer to your patient?

   A. 3.5 mL

   B. 3 mL

   C. 4 mL

   D. 4.3 mL

9. The physician ordered dopamine 7 mcg/kg · min for a patient who weighs 155 lb. The pharmacy delivers dopamine 800 mg in 500 mL D5W. How many milliliters will you administer to your patient per hour?

10. The physician orders for 3000 mL of 1/2 normal saline I.V. that is to be administered over 24 hours. What pump setting will you use?

    A. 124 mL/hr

    B. 120 mL/hr

    C. 125 mL/hr

    D. 126 mL/hr

11. The physician ordered water 1 gal P.O. daily. The patient has an 8-oz cup available at home. How many cups of water should the patient take?

12. The physician ordered 800 mL 1/2 normal saline I.V. over 16 hours. What pump setting will you use?

13. The physician ordered Dilantin 1 mg/kg q6h. The patient weighs 66 lb. The pharmacy delivers Dilantin 15 mg/1 capsule. How many capsule(s) should you administer to your patient?

14. The physician ordered Benadryl 10 mg/kg q6h. The patient weighs 26 lb. The pharmacy delivers Benadryl 125 mg/5 mL. How many milliliters should you administer to your patient?

15. The physician ordered heparin 400 U/hr. The pharmacy delivers 20,000 U heparin in 2000 mL normal saline. How many milliliters will you administer to your patient per hour?

16. The physician ordered dopamine 5 mcg/kg · min for a patient who weighs 185 lb. The pharmacy delivers dopamine 400 mg in 250 D5W. How many milliliters will you administer to the patient per hour?

17. The physician ordered heparin 800 U/hr. The medication label reads 25,000 U heparin in 250 mL D5W. How many milliliters will you administer to your patient per hour?

    A. 7.5 mL
    B. 7 mL
    C. 8 mL
    D. 8.5 mL

18. The physician ordered Zofran 120 mg/kg I.V. The patient weighs 33 lb. The medication label reads 200 mg/mL. You will administer 9 mL to the patient.

    A. True
    B. False

19. The physician ordered Xanax 0.25 mg P.O. daily. The pharmacy delivers Xanax 0.5 mg per tablet. How many tablets to administer to the patient?

20. The physician ordered heparin 400 U/hr. The medication label reads 20,000 U heparin in 400 mL normal saline. How many milliliters will you administer to the patient per hour?

    A. 15 mL
    B. 10 mL
    C. 14 mL
    D. 8 mL

21. The physician ordered Erythromycin 100 mg I.V. The pharmacy delivers Erythromycin 1g/30 mL. How many milliliters will you administer to the patient?

22. The medication order is for 1 L of normal saline I.V. that is to be administered over 8 hours. On hand is I.V. tubing with a 10 gtt/mL drip factor. What is the drip setting?

    A. 21 gtt/min
    B. 2.1 gtt/min
    C. 210 gtt/min
    D. 0.12 gtt/min

23. The physician ordered 350 mL D5W I.V. over 4 hours. What pump setting will you use?

24. The physician ordered Ampicillin 12.5 mg/kg. The patient weighs 40 lb. The pharmacy delivers Ampicillin 100 mg/1 mL. How many milliliters will you administer to the patient?

25. The physician ordered heparin 3000 U S.C. daily. The pharmacy delivers 15,000 U heparin/5 mL. How many milliliters will you administer to the patient?

26. The physician ordered dopamine 6 mcg/kg · min for a patient who weighs 154 lb. The pharmacy delivers dopamine 800 mg in 500 D5W. How many milliliters per hour will you set the infusion pump to?
    A. 15 mL
    B. 16 mL
    C. 14 mL
    D. 17 mL

27. The physician ordered 1 L normal saline I.V. over 12 hours. Use tubing with a 10 gtt/mL drip factor. What is the drip rate?

28. Your patient has received 250 mL of normal saline I.V. and the I.V. bag currently has a volume of 75 mL of normal saline. The pump is set at 30 mL/hr. How much longer does the infusion have to run?
    A. 2 hours 35 minutes
    B. 30 minutes
    C. 2 hours
    D. 2 hours 30 minutes

29. The physician ordered Allopurinol 300 mg P.O. daily. The pharmacy delivers Allopurinol 100 mg per tablet. How many tablets to administer to the patient?

30. The physician ordered 500 mL Ringers Lactate I.V. over 6 hours. Use tubing with a 10 gtt/mL drip factor. What is the drip rate?

31. The physician ordered Benadryl 30 mg/kg · day. The patient weighs 66 lb. The pharmacy delivers Benadryl 125 mg/5 mL. How many milliliters per dose will you administer to the patient?

32. The physician ordered heparin 75 U/hr. The pharmacy delivers 25,000 U heparin in 2000 mL normal saline. How many milliliters will you administer to the patient per hour?

33. The physician ordered heparin 300 U/hr. The pharmacy delivers 20,000 U heparin in 1000 mL D5W. How many milliliters will you administer to the patient per hour?

34. The physician ordered dopamine 3 mcg/kg · min for a patient who weighs 172 lb. The pharmacy delivers dopamine 400 mg in 250mL D5W. How many milliliters will you administer to the patient per hour?

35. The physician ordered dopamine 5 mcg/kg · min for a patient who weighs 200 lb. The pharmacy delivers dopamine 800 mg in 500 D5W. How many milliliters will you administer to the patient per hour?

36. The physician ordered Corophyllin 500 mg q6h PRN. The pharmacy delivers Corophyllin 250 mg/1 rectal suppository. How many suppositories will you administer to the patient?

37. The physician ordered Colace 50 mg P.O. daily. The pharmacy delivers Colace 100 mg per tablet. How many tablets to administer to the patient?

38. The physician ordered Ampicillin 5 mg/kg q6h. The patient weighs 55 lb. The medication label reads 25 mg/mL. What dose will you administer to the patient?

    A. 0.5 mL
    B. 5 mL
    C. 50 mL
    D. 0.05 mL

39. The physician ordered Dilantin 30 mg/kg · day q8h. The patient weighs 55 lb. The pharmacy delivers Dilantin 40 mg/mL. How many milliliters per dose will you administer to the patient?

40. The physician ordered Amoxicillin 10 mg/kg · day q6h. The patient weighs 44 lb. The pharmacy delivers Amoxicillin 125 mg/5 mL. How many milliliters per dose will you administer to the patient?

41. The medication order is for Dilantin 50 mg q6h and the pharmacy delivered Dilantin 125 mg/5 mL. What dose would you administer to the patient?

    A. 5 mL
    B. 4 mL
    C. 3 mL
    D. 2 mL

42. The physician ordered Gentamycin 2 g diluted in 100 mL of normal saline I.V. over 1 hr. Use tubing with a 15 gtt/mL drip factor. What is the drip rate?

43. The physician ordered 100 mL normal saline I.V. over 15 hours. Use tubing with a 15 gtt/mL drip factor. What is the drip rate?

44. The physician ordered Amoxicillin 10 mg/kg. The patient weighs 30 lb. The pharmacy delivers Amoxicillin 125 mg/5 mL. How many milliliters will you administer to the patient?

45. The physician ordered Celocin 6.25 mg/kg q6h. The patient weighs 45 lb. The pharmacy delivers Celocin 75 mg/5 mL. How many milliliters will you administer to the patient?

46. The physician ordered heparin 600 U/hr. The pharmacy delivers 20,000 U heparin in 1000 mL normal saline. How many milliliters will you administer to the patient per hour?

47. The physician ordered heparin 200 U/hr. The medication label reads 20,000 U heparin in 200 mL normal saline. You will administer 2 mL to patient per hour.

   A. True
   B. False

48. The physician ordered dopamine 5 mcg/kg · min for a patient who weighs 187 lb. The pharmacy delivers dopamine 400 mg in 250 D5W. The infusion pump should be set to 16 mL/hour.

   A. True
   B. False

49. The physician ordered dopamine 5 mcg/kg · min for a patient who weighs 175 lb. The pharmacy delivers dopamine 400 mg in 250 D5W. How many milliliters will you administer to the patient per hour?

50. The physician ordered dopamine 7 mcg/kg · min for a patient who weighs 190 lb. The pharmacy delivers dopamine 800 mg in 500 D5W. How many milliliters will you administer to the patient per hour?

51. The physician ordered 25 mL normal saline I.V. over 30 minutes. Use tubing with a 15 gtt/mL drip factor. What is the drip rate?

52. The physician ordered 1000 mL Ringers Lactate I.V. over 12 hours. Use tubing with 15 gtt/mL drip factor. What is the drip rate?

53. The physician ordered Benylin 5 mg/kg P.O. daily. The patient weighs 44 lb. The pharmacy delivers Benylin 50 mg per tablet. How many tablets will you administer to the patient?

54. The physician ordered Lithostat 15 mg/kg P.O. daily. The patient weighs 70 lb. The pharmacy delivers Lithostat 250 mg per tablet. How many tablets will you administer to the patient?

55. The physician ordered Ampicillin 15 mg/kg · day P.O. q8h. The patient weighs 44 lb. The pharmacy delivers Ampicillin 100 mg/mL. How many milliliters per dose will you administer to the patient?

56. The physician ordered Zofran 120 mg/kg · day q6h. The patient weighs 33 lb. The pharmacy delivers Zofran 200 mg/mL. How many milliliters per dose will you administer to the patient?

57. The physician ordered Lithostat 15 mg/kg I.V. daily. The patient weighs 44 lb. The medication label reads 100 mg/mL. What dose will you administer to the patient?
    A. 5 mL
    B. 4 mL
    C. 3 mL
    D. 2 mL

58. The physician ordered Celocin 10 mg/kg · day q6h. The patient weighs 44 lb. The medication label reads 125 mg/5 mL. What dose will you administer to the patient?
    A. 5 mL
    B. 2 mL
    C. 4 mL
    D. 3 mL

59. The medication order is for Cefadyl 10 g diluted in 200 mL of normal saline I.V. that is to be administered over 4 hours. On hand is I.V. tubing with a 15 gtt/mL drip factor. What is the drip setting?
    A. 12 gtt/min
    B. 12.5 gtt/min
    C. 13 gtt/min
    D. 13.5 gtt/min

60. The medication order is for 200 mL of D5W I.V. that is to be administered over 4 hours. The nurse should set the pump at 50 mL/hr.
    A. True
    B. False

61. The physician ordered Capoten 6.25 mg P.O. q8h. The pharmacy delivers Capoten 12.5 mg per tablet. How many tablets to administer to the patient?

62. The physician ordered Morphine Sulfate 2 mg I.M. STAT. The pharmacy delivers Morphine Sulfate 10 mg/mL. How many milliliters to administer to the patient?

63. The physician ordered 1000 mL normal saline I.V. at 40 mL/hr. Use tubing with a 15 gtt/mL drip factor. What is the drip rate?

64. The physician ordered 1000 mL D5W I.V. over 24 hours. What pump setting will you use?

65. The physician ordered 200 mL Lactated Ringers I.V. over 5 hours. What pump setting will you use?

66. The physician ordered Zovirax 5 mg/kg I.V. daily. The patient weighs 30 lb. The pharmacy delivers Zovirax 25 mg/mL. What pump setting will you use?

67. The physician ordered Benylin 25 mg/kg · day I.M. q3h. The patient weighs 55 lb. The pharmacy delivers Benylin 25 mg/mL. How many milliliters per dose will you administer to the patient?

68. The physician ordered heparin 200 U/hr. The pharmacy delivers 25,000 U heparin in 500 mL D5W. How many milliliters will you administer to the patient per hour?

69. The physician ordered heparin 250 U/hr. The pharmacy delivers 25,000 U heparin in 1000 mL D5W. How many milliliters will you administer to the patient per hour?

70. The physician ordered heparin 2500 U S.C. The pharmacy delivers 25,000 U heparin/10 mL. How many milliliters will you administer to the patient?

71. The physician ordered heparin 2000 U S.C. The pharmacy delivers 20,000 U heparin/5 mL. How many milliliters will you administer to the patient?

72. The physician ordered dopamine 7 mcg/kg · min for a patient who weighs 240 lb. The pharmacy delivers dopamine 400 mg in 250 D5W. How many milliliters per hour will you set the infusion pump to?
    A. 28 mL
    B. 29 mL
    C. 28.6 mL
    D. 28.63 mL

73. The physician ordered dopamine 3 mcg/kg · min for a patient who weighs 180 lb. The pharmacy delivers dopamine 400 mg in 250 D5W. How many milliliters per hour will you set the infusion pump to?
    A. 10 mL
    B. 9.20 mL
    C. 9 mL
    D. 9.2 mL

74. The physician ordered Lopid 0.6 g P.O. daily. The pharmacy delivers Lopid 600 mg per tablet. How many tablets will you administer to the patient?

75. The physician ordered Amphojet 5 mL P.O. daily. The patient has a teaspoon available at home. How many teaspoons of the Amphojet should the patient take?

76. The physician ordered 1500 mL Lactated Ringers I.V. over 16 hours. What pump setting will you use?

77. The physician ordered 150 mL D51/2 normal saline I.V. over 5 hours. What pump setting will you use?

78. The physician ordered Zofran 150 mcg/kg I.M. daily. The patient weighs 65 lb. The pharmacy delivers Zofran 2000 mcg/mL. How many milliliters will you administer to the patient?

79. The physician ordered heparin 800 U/hr. The pharmacy delivers 10,000 U heparin in 500 mL normal saline. How many milliliters will you administer to the patient per hour?

80. The physician ordered heparin 400 U/hr. The pharmacy delivers 25,000 U heparin in 2000 mL D5W. How many milliliters will you administer to the patient per hour?

81. The physician ordered dopamine 8 mcg/kg · min for a patient who weighs 220 lb. The pharmacy delivers dopamine 400 mg in 250 D5W. How many milliliters per hour will you set the infusion pump to?

    A. 30 mL
    B. 29.5 mL
    C. 31 mL
    D. 29 mL

82. The physician ordered dopamine 3 mcg/kg · min for a patient who weighs 132 lb. The pharmacy delivers dopamine 400 mg in 250 D5W. How many milliliters per hour will you set the infusion pump to?

    A. 6 mL
    B. 6.2 mL
    C. 6.5 mL
    D. 6.75 mL

83. The physician ordered heparin 7500 U S.C. The pharmacy delivers 20,000 U heparin/2 mL. How many milliliters will you administer to the patient?

84. The physician ordered heparin 8000 U S.C. The pharmacy delivers 20,000 U heparin/10 mL. How many milliliters will you administer to the patient?

85. The physician ordered heparin 100 U/hr. The medication label reads 20,000 U heparin in 2000 mL D5W. How many milliliters will you administer to the patient per hour?

   A. 1 mL
   B. 1.9 mL
   C. 0.9 mL
   D. 10 mL

86. The physician ordered 500 mL D5 1/2 normal saline I.V. over 8 hours. What pump setting will you use?

87. The physician ordered Zovirax 5 mg/kg · day P.O. q12h. The patient weighs 55 lbs. The pharmacy delivers Zovirax 25 mg/tablet. How many tablets per dose will you administer to the patient?

88. The physician ordered Celocin 45 mg/kg · day P.O. q4h. The patient weighs 110 lb. The pharmacy delivers Celocin 125 mg/5 mL. How many milliliters per dose will you administer to the patient?

89. The physician ordered Cephalexin 15 mg/kg · day P.O. q6h. The patient weighs 132 lb. The pharmacy delivers Cephalexin 125 mg/5 mL. How many milliliters per dose will you administer to the patient?

90. The physician ordered heparin 5000 U S.C. The pharmacy delivers 20,000 U heparin/2 mL. How many milliliters will you administer to the patient?

91. The physician ordered heparin 4000 U S.C. The pharmacy delivers 10,000 U heparin/mL. How many milliliters will you administer to the patient?

92. The physician ordered dopamine 8 mcg/kg · min for a patient who weighs 165 lb. The pharmacy delivers dopamine 400 mg in 250 D5W. How many milliliters will you administer to the patient per hour?

93. The physician ordered dopamine 4 mcg/kg · min for a patient who weighs 184 lb. The pharmacy delivers dopamine 400 mg in 250 D5W. How many milliliters will you administer to the patient per hour?

94. The medication order is for Motrin 0.6 g P.O. q6h and the pharmacy delivered Motrin 400 mg per tablet. What dose would you administer to the patient?

   A. 1 tablet
   B. 1.25 tablets
   C. 1.5 tablets
   D. 0.5 tablet

95. The medication order is for Decadron 3 mg P.O. q6h and the pharmacy delivered Decadron 0.75 mg per tablet. What dose would you administer to the patient?

    A. 2.5 tablets
    B. 2 tablets
    C. 4 tablets
    D. 4.5 tablets

96. The physician ordered Methozamine HCl 0.015 g I.M. daily. The pharmacy delivers Methozamine HCl 10 mg/mL. How many milliliters will you administer to the patient?

97. The physician ordered Milk of Magnesia 30 mL P.O. daily. The patient has a tablespoon available at home. How many tablespoons should the patient take of Milk of Magnesia?

98. The physician ordered fruit juice 4000 mL P.O. daily. The patient has a 1-qt container available at home. How many quarts should the patient take of fruit juice?

99. The medication order is for 600 mL of 1/2 normal saline I.V. that is to be administered over 6 hours. On hand is I.V. tubing with a 10 gtt/mL drip factor. What pump setting will you use?

    A. 15 gtt/min
    B. 16 gtt/min
    C. 17 gtt/min
    D. 18 gtt/min

100. The physician ordered Cephalexin 15 mg/kg P.O. daily. The patient weighs 45 lb. The pharmacy delivers Cephalexin 125 mg/5 mL. How many milliliters will you administer to the patient?

CORRECT ANSWERS AND RATIONALES

1. 10 gtt/min
2. 2 tablets
3. C. 1.75 mL
4. 4 mL
5. 23 mL/hr
6. D. 0.5 mL
7. 125 mL
8. A. 3.5 mL

9. 18.5 mL
10. C. 125 mL/hr
11. 16 cups
12. 50 mL
13. 2 capsules
14. 4.7 mL
15. 40 mL
16. 16 mL/hr

17. C. 8 mL
18. A. True
19. 0.5 tablet
20. D. 8 mL
21. 3 mL
22. A. 21 gtt/min
23. 88 mL
24. 2.3 mL

25. 1 mL
26. B. 16 mL
27. 14 gtt/min
28. D. 2 hours 30 minutes
29. 3 tablet
30. 14 gtt/min
31. 36 mL
32. 6 mL
33. 15 mL
34. 9 mL/hr
35. 17 mL/hr
36. 2 rectal suppositories
37. 0.5 tablet
38. B. 5 mL
39. 6.25 mL
40. 2 mL
41. D. 2 mL
42. 25 gtt/min
43. 2 gtt/min
44. 5 mL
45. 8.5 mL
46. 30 mL
47. A. True
48. A. True
49. 15 mL/hr
50. 23 mL/hr
51. 13 gtt/min
52. 21 gtt/min
53. 2 tablets
54. 2 tablets
55. 1 mL
56. 2.25 mL
57. C. 3 mL
58. B. 2 mL
59. C. 13 gtt/min
60. A. True
61. 0.5 tablet
62. 0.2 mL
63. 10 gtt/min
64. 42 mL
65. 40 mL
66. 2.7 mL
67. 3 mL
68. 4 mL
69. 10 mL
70. 1 mL
71. 0.5 mL
72. B. 29 mL
73. C. 9 mL
74. 1 tablet
75. 1 teaspoon
76. 94 mL
77. 30 mL
78. 2.2 mL
79. 40 mL
80. 32 mL
81. A. 30 mL
82. D. 6.75 mL
83. 0.75 mL
84. 4 mL
85. D. 10 mL
86. 62.5 mL
87. 2.5 tablets
88. 15 mL
89. 9 mL
90. 0.5 mL
91. 0.4 mL
92. 22 mL/hr
93. 12.5 mL/hr
94. C. 1.5 tablets
95. C. 4 tablets
96. 1.5 mL
97. 2 tablespoons
98. 4 qt
99. C. 17 gtt/min
100. 12 mL

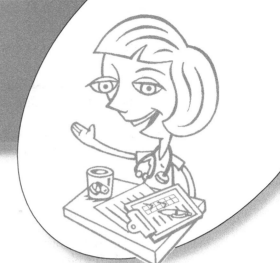

Final Exam Part 2

1. The medication order is for 2 L of normal saline I.V. that is to be administered over 16 hours. On hand is I.V. tubing with a 15 gtt/mL drip factor. What is the drip setting?

   A. 31 gtt/min
   B. 3.1 gtt/min
   C. 310 gtt/min
   D. 0.31 gtt/min

2. The medication order is for Dilantin 75 mg and the pharmacy delivered Dilantin 150 mg/2 mL. What dose would you administer to the patient?

   A. 2 mL
   B. 1.5 mL
   C. 1 mL
   D. 2.5 mL

3. Your patient has received 500 mL of Sodium Chloride I.V. and the I.V. bag currently has a volume of 50 mL of Sodium Chloride. The pump is set at 20 mL/hr. How much longer does the infusion have to run?

   A. 2 hours 5 minutes
   B. 30 minutes
   C. 2 hours
   D. 2 hours 30 minutes

4. The physician ordered 500 mL Ringers Lactate I.V. over 24 hours. Use microdrip tubing. What is the drip rate?

5. The physician ordered Erythromycin 200 mg I.V. The pharmacy delivers Erythromycin 2 g/60 mL. How many milliliters will you administer to the patient?

6. The physician ordered dopamine 5 mcg/kg · min for a patient who weighs 125 lb. The pharmacy delivers dopamine 800 mg in 500 D5W. How many milliliters will you administer to your patient per hour?

7. The physician ordered dopamine 6 mcg/kg · min for a patient who weighs 150 lb. The pharmacy delivers dopamine 800 mg in 500 D5W. How many milliliters will you administer to the patient per hour?

8. The medication order is for Cefadyl 50 g diluted in 300 mL of normal saline I.V. that is to be administered over 8 hours. On hand is I.V. tubing with a 10 gtt/mL drip factor. What is the drip setting?

   A. 6 gtt/min
   B. 6.5 gtt/min
   C. 7 gtt/min
   D. 7.5 gtt/min

9. The physician ordered heparin 4000 U S.C. The pharmacy delivers 20,000 U heparin/150 mL. How many milliliters will you administer to the patient?

10. The physician ordered dopamine 4 mcg/kg · min for a patient who weighs 175 lb. The pharmacy delivers dopamine 800 mg in 500 D5W. How many milliliters will you administer to the patient per hour?

11. The physician ordered Corophyllin 500 mg q8h PRN. The pharmacy delivers Corophyllin 250 mg/rectal suppository. How many rectal suppositories to administer to the patient?

12. The physician ordered Heparin 800 U/hr. The medication label reads 20,000 U heparin in 600 mL normal saline. How many milliliters will you administer to the patient per hour?

   A. 25 mL
   B. 20 mL
   C. 24 mL
   D. 23 mL

13. The physician ordered Ampicillin 20 mg/kg. The patient weighs 157 lb. The medication label reads 50 mg/mL. What dose will you administer to your patient?

   A. 28.5 mL
   B. 28 mL

C. 29 mL

D. 29.5 mL

14. The physician ordered Amoxicillin 30 mg/kg. The patient weighs 66 lb. The pharmacy delivers Amoxicillin 250 mg/10 mL. How many milliliters will you administer to the patient?

15. The physician ordered dopamine 6 mcg/kg · min for a patient who weighs 280 lb. The pharmacy delivers dopamine 800 mg in 500 mL D5W. How many milliliters per hour will you set the infusion pump?

    A. 27 mL

    B. 27.5 mL

    C. 29 mL

    D. 28.6 mL

16. The physician ordered 150 mL D5 1/2 normal saline I.V. over 2 hours. What pump setting will you use?

17. The physician ordered Milk of Magnesia 15 mL P.O. q.i.d. The patient has a tablespoon available at home. How many tablespoons of Milk of Magnesia should the patient take?

18. The physician ordered Morphine Sulfate 32 mg I.M. STAT. The pharmacy delivers Morphine Sulfate 15 mg/mL. How many milliliters will you administer to the patient?

19. The physician ordered Gentamycin 4 g diluted in 200 mL of normal saline I.V. over 2 hours. Use tubing with a 10 gtt/mL drip factor. What is the drip rate?

20. The physician ordered 650 mL D5W I.V. over 8 hours. What pump setting will you use?

21. The physician orders are for 250 mL of 1/2 normal saline I.V. that is to be administered over 12 hours. What pump setting will you use?

    A. 20.75 mL/hr

    B. 20 mL/hr

    C. 20.8 mL/hr

    D. 20.7 mL/hr

22. The physician ordered 500 mL of 0.9% of normal saline I.V. over 30 mL/hr. On hand is tubing with a 15 gtt/mL drip factor. What drip rate would you use?

23. The physician ordered Ampicillin 15 mg/kg. The patient weighs 80 lb. The pharmacy delivers Ampicillin 200 mg/mL. How many milliliters will you administer to the patient?

24. The physician ordered Celocin 3.25 mg/kg. The patient weighs 75 lb. The pharmacy delivers Celocin 50 mg/5 mL. How many milliliters will you administer to the patient?

25. The physician ordered Zofran 140 mg/kg · day q8h. The patient weighs 77 lb. The pharmacy delivers Zofran 250 mg/mL. How many milliliters per dose will you administer to the patient?

26. The physician ordered 2000 mL normal saline I.V. at 20 mL/hr. Use tubing with a 15 gtt/mL drip factor. What is the drip rate?

27. The physician ordered dopamine 5 mcg/kg · min for a patient who weighs 340 lb. The pharmacy delivers dopamine 400 mg in 250 D5W. How many milliliters per hour will you set the infusion pump?
    A. 28 mL
    B. 29 mL
    C. 28.6 mL
    D. 28.63 mL

28. The physician ordered heparin 200 U/hr. The pharmacy delivers 25,000 U heparin in 4000-mL D5W. How many milliliters will you administer to the patient per hour?

29. The physician ordered heparin 4000 U S.C. The pharmacy delivers 25,000 U heparin/800 mL. How many milliliters will you administer to the patient?

30. The physician ordered heparin 600 U/hr. The pharmacy delivers 15,000 U heparin in 500-mL normal saline. How many milliliters will you administer to the patient per hour?

31. The physician ordered Zovirax 2mg/kg · day q12h. The patient weighs 160 lb. The pharmacy delivers Zovirax 50 mg per tablet. How many tablets per dose will you administer to the patient?

32. The physician ordered Benylin 25 mg/kg. The patient weighs 88 lb. The pharmacy delivers Benylin 75 mg per tablet. How many tablets will you administer to the patient?

33. The physician ordered Gentamycin 0.55 mg P.O. q.i.d. The pharmacy delivers Gentamycin 0.75 mg per 2 tablets. How many tablets will you administer to the patient?

34. The physician ordered dopamine 10 mcg/kg · min for a patient who weighs 170 lb. The pharmacy delivers dopamine 800 mg in 500 D5W. How many milliliters will you administer to your patient per hour?

35. The physician ordered Zofran 100 mg/kg. The patient weighs 75 lb. The medication label reads 250 mg/mL. You will administer 15 mL to the patient.

    A. True

    B. False

36. The physician ordered heparin 6000 U S.C. The medication label reads 20,000 U heparin/100 mL. How many milliliters will you administer to the patient per hour?

    A. 30.25 mL

    B. 30 mL

    C. 30.75 mL

    D. 40 mL

37. The physician ordered Benadryl 35 mg/kg · day q12h. The patient weighs 82 lb. The pharmacy delivers Benadryl 250 mg/10 mL. How many milliliters per dose will you administer to the patient?

38. The physician ordered Heparin 25,000 U/hr. The medication label reads 20,000 U heparin in 3000 mL normal saline. You will administer 5 mL/hr to the patient.

    A. True

    B. False

39. The physician ordered Amphojet 15 mL P.O. q.i.d. The patient has a teaspoon available at home. How many teaspoons will the patient require to administer Amphojet 15 mL?

40. The physician ordered heparin 1000 U S.C. The pharmacy delivers 20,000 U heparin/700 mL. How many milliliters will you administer to the patient?

41. The physician ordered Cephalexin 10 mg/kg. The patient weighs 145 lb. The pharmacy delivers Cephalexin 125 mg/8 mL. How many milliliters will you administer to the patient?

42. The medication order is for 500 mL of D5W I.V. that is to be administered over 8 hours. The nurse should set the pump at 75 mL/hr.

    A. True

    B. False

43. The physician ordered heparin 300 U/hr. The pharmacy delivers 25,000 U heparin in 800 mL D5W. How many milliliters will you administer to the patient per hour?

44. The physician ordered Benylin 15 mg/kg. The patient weighs 30 lb. The pharmacy delivers Benylin 50 mg per tablet. How many tablets will you administer to the patient?

45. The physician ordered Ampicillin 15 mg/kg. The patient weighs 45 lb. The pharmacy delivers Ampicillin 250 mg/10 mL. How many milliliters should you administer to your patient?

46. The physician ordered Dilantin 60 mg/kg · day q4h. The patient weighs 130 lb. The pharmacy delivers Dilantin 125 mg/mL. How many milliliters per dose will you administer to your patient?

47. The physician ordered Ampicillin 75 mg. The patient weighs 95 lb. The medication label reads 50 mg/mL. What dose will you administer to the patient?

    A. 1.5 mL
    B. 0.15 mL
    C. 50 mL
    D. 0.05 mL

48. The physician ordered Celocin 20 mg/kg · day q6h. The patient weighs 125 lb. The medication label reads 175 mg/5 mL. What dose will you administer to the patient?

    A. 8.1 mL
    B. 8.2 mL
    C. 8 mL
    D. 7.5 mL

49. The physician ordered heparin 3500 U S.C. The pharmacy delivers 25,000 U heparin/200 mL. How many milliliters will you administer to the patient?

50. The physician ordered heparin 7000 U S.C. The pharmacy delivers 20,000 U heparin/300 mL. How many milliliters will you administer to the patient?

51. The medication order is for Motrin 0.8 g and the pharmacy delivered Motrin 400 mg per tablet. What dose would you administer to the patient?

    A. 1 tablet
    B. 1.25 tablets
    C. 1.5 tablets
    D. 2 tablets

52. The physician ordered Lithostat 6 mg/kg. The patient weighs 150 lb. The pharmacy delivers Lithostat 150 mg per tablet. How many tablets will you administer to the patient?

53. The physician ordered Dilantin 15 mg/kg · day q8h. The patient weighs 150 lb. The pharmacy delivers Dilantin 20 mg/mL. How many milliliters per dose will you administer to the patient?

54. The physician ordered Benadryl 2 mg/kg. The patient weighs 88 lb. The pharmacy delivers Benadryl 25 mg/1 capsule. How many capsule(s) will you administer to the patient?

55. The physician ordered Zovirax 200 mg P.O. q.i.d. The pharmacy delivers Zovirax 0.1 g per tablet. How many tablets would you administer to your patient?

56. The physician ordered dopamine 12 mcg/kg · min for a patient who weighs 170 lb. The pharmacy delivers dopamine 800 mg in 500 D5W. How many milliliters per hour will you set the infusion pump?

    A. 32.2 mL
    B. 30 mL
    C. 34.8 mL
    D. 35 mL

57. The physician ordered Amoxicillin 20 mg/kg · day q6h. The patient weighs 97 lb. The pharmacy delivers Amoxicillin 125 mg/10 mL. How many milliliters per dose will you administer to the patient?

58. The physician ordered Zovirax 8 mg/kg. The patient weighs 45 lb. The pharmacy delivers Zovirax 25 mg/mL. How many milliliters per dose will you administer to the patient?

59. The physician ordered dopamine 2 mcg/kg · min for a patient who weighs 120 lb. The pharmacy delivers dopamine 400 mg in 250 mL D5W. How many milliliters per hour will you set the infusion pump?

60. The physician ordered dopamine 10 mcg/kg · min for a patient who weighs 85 lb. The pharmacy delivers dopamine 400 mg in 250 mL D5W. How many milliliters will you administer to the patient per hour?

61. The physician ordered Benylin 15 mg/kg · day q3h. The patient weighs 75 lb. The pharmacy delivers Benylin 50 mg/1 mL. How many milliliters per dose will you administer to the patient?

62. The physician ordered dopamine 15 mcg/kg · min for a patient that weighs 194 lb. The pharmacy delivers dopamine 800 mg in 500 mL D5W. The infusion pump should be set to 15 mL/hr.

    A. True
    B. False

63. The physician ordered heparin 500 U/hr. The pharmacy delivers 20,000 U heparin in 2000-mL D5W. How many milliliters will you administer to the patient per hour?

64. The physician ordered dopamine 35 mcg/kg · min for a patient who weighs 125 lb. The pharmacy delivers dopamine 400 mg in 250 D5W. How many milliliters will you administer to the patient per hour?

65. The physician ordered Capoten 3 mg P.O. q8h. The pharmacy delivers Capoten 6 mg per tablet. How many tablets will you administer to the patient?

66. The physician ordered 250 mL D5 1/2 normal saline I.V. over 6 hours. What pump setting will you use?

67. The physician ordered dopamine 6 mcg/kg · min for a patient who weighs 284 lb. The pharmacy delivers dopamine 800 mg in 500 D5W. How many milliliters will you administer to the patient per hour?

68. The medication order is for 900 mL of 1/2 normal saline I.V. that is to be administered over 8 hours. On hand is I.V. tubing with a 15 gtt/mL drip factor. What pump setting will you use?

   A. 112.5 mL/hr
   B. 111 mL/hr
   C. 100 mL/hr
   D. 112 mL/hr

69. The physician ordered Zofran 250 mcg/kg. The patient weighs 165 lb. The pharmacy delivers Zofran 4000 mcg/mL. How many milliliters will you administer to the patient?

   A. 4 mL
   B. 4.7 mL
   C. 3.7 mL
   D. 3 mL

70. The physician ordered Ampicillin 25 mg/kg · day q8h. The patient weighs 65 lb. The pharmacy delivers Ampicillin 125 mg/mL. How many milliliters per dose will you administer to the patient?

71. The physician ordered 750 mL Ringers Lactate I.V. over 18 hour. Use tubing with a 10 gtt/mL drip factor. What is the drip rate?

72. The physician ordered Heparin 1000 U/hr. The medication label reads 25,000 U heparin in 250 mL D5W. How many milliliters will you administer to your patient per hour?

   A. 10 mL
   B. 12 mL
   C. 13 mL
   D. 12.5 mL

73. The physician ordered 250 mL Sodium Chloride I.V. over 18 hours. What pump setting would you use?

74. The physician ordered Allopurinol 250 mg P.O. q.i.d. The pharmacy delivers Allopurinol 150 mg per 2 tablets. How many tablets to administer to the patient?

75. The physician ordered 50 mL normal saline I.V. over 30 minutes. Use tubing with a 10 gtt/mL drip factor. What is the drip rate?

76. The physician ordered Lopid 0.8 g P.O. q.i.d. The pharmacy delivers Lopid 800 mg per tablet. How many tablets to administer to the patient?

77. The physician ordered Heparin 250 U/hr. The medication label reads 20,000 U heparin in 4000 mL D5W. How many milliliters will you administer to the patient per hour?
    A. 52 mL
    B. 51 mL
    C. 50 mL
    D. 49 mL

78. The medication order is for Decadron 2 mg and the pharmacy delivered Decadron 0.50 mg per tablet. What dose would you administer to the patient?
    A. 2.5 tablets
    B. 2 tablets
    C. 4 tablets
    D. 4.5 tablets

79. The physician ordered 2000 mL D5W I.V. over 16 hours. What pump setting will you use?

80. The physician ordered heparin 800 U/hr. The pharmacy delivers 20,000 U heparin in 2000 mL normal saline. How many milliliters will you administer to the patient per hour?

81. The physician ordered 1600 mL 1/2 sodium chloride I.V. over 18 hours. What pump setting will you use?

82. The physician ordered dopamine 9 mcg/kg · min for a patient who weighs 125 lb. The pharmacy delivers dopamine 400 mg in 250 D5W. How many milliliters will you administer to your patient per hour?

83. The physician orders for Xanax 35 mg and the pharmacy delivered Xanax 75 mg/5 mL. What dose would you administer to the patient?

    A. 0.22 mL

    B. 0.25 mL

    C. 0.3 mL

    D. 0 mL

84. The physician ordered 3000 mL normal saline I.V. over 24 hours. Use tubing with a 10 gtt/mL drip factor. What is the drip rate?

85. The physician ordered 2500 mL Lactated Ringers I.V. over 24 hours. What pump setting will you use?

86. The physician ordered Celocin 15 mg/kg · day q8h. The patient weighs 210 lb. The pharmacy delivers Celocin 125 mg/2 mL. How many milliliters per dose will you administer to the patient?

87. The physician ordered fruit juice 2000 mL P.O. q.i.d. The patient has a 1-qt container available at home. How many quarts should the patient take of fruit juice?

88. The physician ordered heparin 800 U S.C. The pharmacy delivers 25,000 U heparin/500 mL. How many milliliters will you administer to the patient?

89. The physician ordered heparin 350 U S.C. The pharmacy delivers 15,000 U heparin/200 mL. How many milliliters will you administer to the patient?

90. The physician ordered heparin 600 U/hr. The pharmacy delivers 15,000 U heparin in 1000 mL normal saline. How many milliliters will you administer to your patient per hour?

91. The physician ordered Colace 400 mg P.O. q.i.d. The pharmacy delivers Colace 200 mg/1 capsule. How many milliliters you will administer to the patient?

92. The physician ordered heparin 500 U/hr. The pharmacy delivers 25,000 U heparin in 2000 mL D5W. How many milliliters will you administer to the patient per hour?

93. The physician ordered dopamine 6 mcg/kg · min for a patient who weighs 232 lb. The pharmacy delivers dopamine 400 mg in 250 D5W. How many milliliters per hour will you set the infusion pump?

    A. 23.5 mL

    B. 23 mL

    C. 23.8 mL

    D. 23.7 mL

94. The physician ordered Cephalexin 10 mg/kg · day q8h. The patient weighs 232 lb. The pharmacy delivers Cephalexin 250 mg/5 mL. How many milliliters per dose will you administer to the patient?

95. The physician ordered dopamine 15 mcg/kg · min for a patient who weighs 250 lb. The pharmacy delivers dopamine 800 mg in 500 D5W. How many milliliters will you administer to the patient per hour?

96. The physician ordered Lithostat 5 mg/kg. The patient weighs 85 lb. the medication label reads 150 mg/mL. What dose will you administer to the patient?

    A. 1.55 mL
    B. 1.4 mL
    C. 1.3 mL
    D. 1.2 mL

97. The physician ordered GoLytely 1 gal P.O. q.i.d. The patient has a 12-oz cup available at home. How many cups of GoLytely should the patient take?

98. The physician ordered 400 mL Lactated Ringers I.V. over 8 hours. What pump setting will you use?

99. The physician ordered heparin 50 U/hr. The pharmacy delivers 25,000 U heparin in 3000 mL normal saline. How many milliliters will you administer to the patient per hour?

100. The physician ordered Methozamine HCl 0.025 g I.M. q.i.d. The pharmacy delivers Methozamine HCl 20 mg/mL. How many milliliters will you administer to the patient?

CORRECT ANSWERS AND RATIONALES

1. A. 31 gtt/min
2. C. 1 mL
3. D. 2 hours 30 minutes
4. 21 gtt/min
5. 6 mL
6. 10.7 mL
7. 15.3 mL/hr
8. B. 6.5 gtt/min
9. 30 mL
10. 11.9 mL/hr
11. 2 rectal suppositories
12. C. 24 mL
13. A. 28.5 mL
14. 36 mL
15. D. 28.6 mL
16. 75 mL
17. 1 tablespoon
18. 2.1 mL
19. 7 gtt/min
20. 81.25 mL/hr
21. C. 20.8 mL/hr
22. 8 gtt/min
23. 2.7 mL
24. 11 mL
25. 6.5 mL
26. 5 gtt/min
27. B. 29 mL
28. 32 mL
29. 128 mL
30. 20 mL
31. 1.5 tablets

32. 13 tablets
33. 0.5 tablet
34. 29 mL/hr
35. B. False
36. B. 30 mL
37. 26 mL
38. B. False
39. 3 teaspoons
40. 2 mL
41. 42.2 mL
42. B. False
43. 9.6 mL/hr
44. 4 tablets
45. 12.3 mL
46. 4.7 mL
47. A. 1.5 mL
48. A. 8.1 mL
49. 28 mL
50. 105 mL
51. D. 2 tablets
52. 3 mL
53. 17 mL
54. 3 capsules

55. 2 tablets
56. C. 34.8 mL
57. 17.6 mL
58. 6.5 mL
59. 4.1 mL/hr
60. 14.5 mL/hr
61. 1.3 mL
62. B. False
63. 50 mL/hr
64. 74.6 mL/hr
65. 0.5 tablet
66. 41.7 mL/hr
67. 29 mL/hr
68. A. 112.5 mL/hr
69. B. 4.7 mL
70. 2 mL
71. 6.9 gtt/min
72. A. 10 mL
73. 13.9 mL/hr
74. 3 tablets
75. 17 gtt/min
76. 1 tablet
77. C. 50 mL

78. C. 4 tablets
79. 125 mL/hr
80. 80 mL/hr
81. 88.9 mL/hr
82. 19.2 mL/hr
83. A. 0.22 mL
84. 20.8 gtt/min
85. 104.2 mL/hr
86. 7.6 mL
87. 2 qt
88. 16 mL
89. 4.7 mL
90. 40 mL/hr
91. 2 capsules
92. 40 mL/hr
93. D. 23.7 mL
94. 7 mL
95. 63.9 mL/hr
96. C. 1.3 mL
97. 11 cups
98. 50 mL/hr
99. 6 mL/hr
100. 1.25 mL

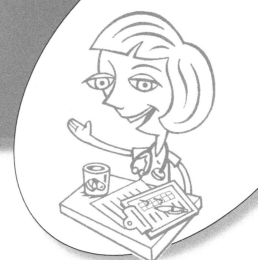

Final Exam Part 3

1. The fraction of the patients on the psychiatric unit going to off-unit recreation is 3/5. During recreation 1/3 of those patients play computer games. What fraction of the patients plays computer games during recreation?

   A. 1/5
   B. 2/5
   C. 2/3
   D. 1/3

2. The pharmacy sent four tablets each containing 12.5 mg of medication. What is the total dose given to the patient if you administered all four tablets?

   A. 12.5 mg
   B. 50 mg
   C. 25 mg
   D. 24 mg

3. Emergency Medical Services (EMS) has a choice of two health care facilities. One is 7.3 miles from the patient's home and the other is 8.4 miles from the patient's home. How much future away from the patient's home is the second health care facility?

   A. 1 mile
   B. 3.4 miles
   C. 1.1 miles
   D. 2.1 miles

4. The nurse assessed 2/5 of the patients. What fraction of the patients is left to be assessed?

   A. 3/5

   B. 1/5

   C. 2/5

   D. 4/5

5. A patient ate 1/2 of breakfast when he awaken and then 1/6 of his breakfast before noon. What fraction of his breakfast did he eat?

   A. 1/6

   B. 5/6

   C. 2/6

   D. 4/6

6. The patient drank 1.4 oz of juice, 12.7 oz of water, and 0.4 oz of milk. How many oz of fluid did the patient receive?

   A. 14 oz

   B. 24 oz

   C. 14.3 oz

   D. 14.5 oz

7. The West Wing unit has 30 patients. The East Wing unit has 0.2 as many patients. How many patients are in the West Wing?

   A. 6 patients

   B. 4 patients

   C. 7.5 patients

   D. 6.5 patients

8. A patient is receiving 1000 L of I.V. fluid at 166.67 L/hr. Approximately how many hours for the 1000 L to infuse into the patient?

   A. 8 hours

   B. 5 hours

   C. 6 hours

   D. 7 hours

9. Of a pie, 2/4 remains. You want to divide the remaining equally between two patients. How much does each patient receive?

   A. 1/8

   B. 1/16

   C. 2/8

   D. 2/5

10. The nurse takes 5.5 minutes to administer medication to a patient. The nurse has nine patients. How many minutes will it take the nurse to administer medication to all patients?

    A. 49.5 minutes
    B. 50 minutes
    C. 50.1 minutes
    D. 49.8 minutes

11. A new nurse took 10.7 minutes per patient to medicate his patients. After a year, he takes 8.3 minutes per patients. How many fewer minutes does the nurse require to administer medication?

    A. 3.4 minutes
    B. 2.4 minutes
    C. 1.5 minutes
    D. 3.6 minutes

12. $(-7) \times (-3) =$

13. What percent is 20 of 180?

14. $1.86 \div 0.6 =$

15. $4/9 \div 4/5 =$

16. A patient who had knee surgery was placed on a continuous passive motion (CPM) device that mechanically manipulates the patient's leg. The fully extended leg is measured as 0 degrees. The CPM device bends the knee measured as less than 0 degrees, which is a negative number. At the beginning of the week, the patient knee moved −8 degrees. At the end of the week, the patient was able to move his knee −16 degrees. What distance has the knee moved over the week?

    A. 9 degrees
    B. 19 degrees
    C. (−19 degrees)
    D. (−9 degrees)

17. $(-15) \div (-5) =$

18. A bag of normal saline contains 1000 L. The practitioner order 250 L/hr. How many hours will it take to infuse 1000 L?

    A. 4 hours
    B. 6 hours
    C. 12 hours
    D. 5 hours

19. $x: 64 = 1: 32; x =$

20. The patients ate a tray of baked ziti and had 1/3 the tray left over. The next day the patients ate 2/3 of what was left. The patients ate the remaining baked ziti on the third day. How much baked ziti did patients eat on the third day?

    A. 1/5
    B. 2/9
    C. 1/4
    D. 1/3

21. There are 98 patients. The nurse manager uses 1 nurse to 8 patients ratio and 1 CNA to 12 patients. Write an expression that shows the relationship between patients, nurses, CNAs, and the total number of clinical staff (nurse and CNAs) required to care for patients?

    A. $98 \times 8 \times 12$ = Total Number of Clinical Staff
    B. (Number of Patients/8) + (Number of Patients/12) = Total Number of Clinical Staff
    C. $98 + 8 + 12$ = Total Number of Clinical Staff
    D. (Number of Patients $\times$ 8) $\times$ (Number of Patients $\times$ 12) = Total Number of Clinical Staff

22. $5/8 \times 1/4 =$

23. A patient with liver failure underwent paracentesis for ascites. Fluid removed each day is 3 L. How many liters were removed in the past 4 days?

    A. 5 liters
    B. 1.3 liters
    C. 8 liters
    D. 1.5 liters

24. $82 - x = (5 + 10)$

25. Write an expression that shows the following relationship. Total time needed to administer medication for all patients on the day shift is the sum of the time spent on each medication pass. The nurse spends 30 minutes per patient administering morning medications; 20 minutes per patient administering noon medications; 15 minutes per patient administering 2 PM medications; and 2 minutes per patient during the shift administering PRN medication.

    A. (Number of Patients/30 min) + (Number of Patients/20 min) + (Number of Patients/15 min) + (Number of Patients/2 min) = Total Time to Administer Medication to All Patients on the Day Shift
    B. (Number of Patients + 30 min) $\times$ (Number of Patients + 20 min) $\times$ (Number of Patients + 15 min) $\times$ (Number of Patients + 2 min) = Total Time to Administer Medication to All Patients on the Day shift

C. (Number of Patients + 30 min) + (Number of Patients + 20 min) + (Number of Patients + 15 min) + (Number of Patients + 2 min) = Total Time to Administer Medication to All Patients on the Day shift

D. (Number of Patients × 30 min) + (Number of Patients × 20 min) + (Number of Patients × 15 min) + (Number of Patients × 2 min) = Total Time to Administer Medication to All Patients on the Day Shift

26. $0.225 \div 4 =$

27. A patient who is recovering from a stroke undergoes physical therapy to help regain his ability to ambulate. The therapist measures the number of footsteps the patient takes regardless of the direction. In each of the four attempts, the patient took five steps backwards. The therapist recorded this as $(-5) \times 4 =$. How many steps did the patient take?

A. 13 steps
B. 20 steps
C. (−13 steps)
D. (−20 steps)

28. What percent is 52 of 224?

29. $y \times 8 = 16$

30. $3 : x = 1 : 6; x =$

31. $7 - (-3) =$

32. The health care facility has a ratio of 1 CNA:2 nurses and a ratio of 1 nurse: 8 patients. Your unit has 32 patients. How many CNAs would you schedule?

A. 5 CNAs
B. 4 CNAs
C. 3 CNAs
D. 2 CNAs

33. The nurse manager wrote the following equation but forgot to label values in the equation. You are told to calculate the equation to determine the number of juice boxes that are expected to be delivered by dietary. How many boxes of juice will be delivered?

$$10 \times 4 + 2 = \text{Total boxes of juice}$$

A. 80
B. 42
C. 60
D. 62

34. The children's unit at the hospital encourages young patients to eat meals by awarding points that can be redeemed once a day for a prize. Failure to eat meals causes the young patient to lose points. Six-year-old Bob received 12 points before lunch. He told the nurse that he ate all his lunch. The nurse awarded Bob 5 points bringing Bob's total to 17 points. However, the CNA told the nurse Bob did not eat all his lunch. The nurse deducted points using the following expression: $17 - (+7) =$. This states that a positive 7 points are being removed from the total points. What is the result of this expression?

   A. 15

   B. 20

   C. 10

   D. 5

35. A patient weight 118 lb. The practitioner orders a diet that will increase the patient's weight by 1.2 during the patient stay in the hospital. What is the patient's weight goal?

   A. 110.5 lb

   B. 110 lb

   C. 141.1 lb

   D. 141.5 lb

36. $3/8 \div 4/5 =$

37. $0.33 \times 0.32 =$

38. What percent is 27 of 82?

39. $x:30 = 1:5; x =$

40. $(4 \times 5) + (6 - 3) \times 2 =$

41. The health care facility developed a formula for determining CNA staffing levels. The expression is used to describe the relationships among the number of patients, CNA assignment, and required number of CNAs. How many CNAs are required for 25 patients and a CNA assignment of 0.2?

   Number of Patients $\times$ CNA Assignment = Required Number of CNAs

   A. 5 CNAs

   B. 4 CNAs

   C. 2 CNAs

   D. 6 CNAs

42. Refer to the expression in problem 41. If the nurse manager scheduled 5 CNAs, how many patients are on the unit?

A. 32 patients
B. 30 patients
C. 50 patients
D. 25 patients

43. The dietician uses the ratio of 2 hamburgers:1 patient. Your unit has 25 patients. How many hamburgers do you expect to receive?

    A. 26 hamburgers
    B. 50 hamburgers
    C. 46 hamburgers
    D. 16 hamburgers

44. x:36 = 1:9; x =

45. x:24 = 2:16; x =

46. 9 − (−7) =

47. A patient was given range of motion exercise for her arm. Holding her arm straight in front of her is considered 0 degrees. Raising her arm is considered positive degrees and lowering her arm is considered negative degrees. She lowered her arm 6 degrees on Monday and 18 degrees on Tuesday. How many degrees in total did she move her arm?

    A. 24 degrees
    B. (−24 degrees)
    C. (−5 degrees)
    D. 5 degrees

48. By Friday, the patient in question 47 was able to lower her arm 30 degrees. How much movement since Monday she did?

    A. (−37 degrees)
    B. 37 degrees
    C. (−24 degrees)
    D. (−10 degrees)

49. Staffing requirements for nurses is based on the acuity of the patient. The acuity is assessed by the patient's diagnosis, which reflects the amount of time the nurse will likely spend per shift caring for the patient. For an average patient the acuity factor is 1. For an unstable patient the acuity factor is 2 and for a critically ill patient the acuity factor is 4. The acuity factor is divided into the normal eight patient assignment per nurse to determine the number of patients per nurse is assigned. Write the expression that shows this relationship between the number of critically ill patients that will be assigned to a nurse.

    A. 4/8 = number of patients per nurse

    B. 8/4 = number of patients per nurse

    C. 2/8 = number of patients per nurse

    D. 8/2 = number of patients per nurse

50. **Based on problem 49, write an equation that determines the number of nurses required to care for 20 average patients, 16 unstable patients, and 8 critically ill patients.**

    A. $(20 + (8/1)) + (16 + (8/2)) + (8 + (8/4)) = $ Total Number of Nurses

    B. $(20/(8/1)) + (16/(8/2)) + (8/(8/4)) = $ Total Number of Nurses

    C. $(20 + (8/1)) \times (16 + (8/2)) \times (8 + (8/4)) = $ Total Number of Nurses

    D. $(20 \times (8/1)) \times (16 \times (8/2)) \times (8 \times (8/4)) = $ Total Number of Nurses

51. **Fraction of the patients on the pediatric unit going to recreation is 1/5. During recreation 2/3 of those patients draw pictures for their parents. What fraction of the patients draw pictures for their parents during recreation?**

    A. 2/5

    B. 1/15

    C. 2/3

    D. 1/3

52. **The pharmacy sent 3 tablets each containing 26.2 mg of medication. What is the total dose given to the patient if you administered all four tablets?**

    A. 12.5 mg

    B. 78.6 mg

    C. 25.6 mg

    D. 78 mg

53. **EMS has a choice of two health care facilities. One is 6.3 miles from the patient's home and the other is 9.2 miles from the patient's home. How much future away from the patient's home is the second health care facility?**

    A. 1 mile

    B. 9.4 miles

    C. 9.2 miles

    D. 9.1 miles

54. **The nurse assessed 3/8 of the patients. What fraction of the patients is left to be assessed?**

    A. 5/8

    B. 1/8

    C. 2/8

    D. 4/8

55. A patient ate 1/4 of breakfast when he awaken and then 1/5 of his breakfast before noon. What fraction of his breakfast did he eat?

    A. 1/6
    B. 5/6
    C. 2/16
    D. 9/20

56. The patient drank 1.2 oz of juice, 11.5 oz of water, and 0.8 oz of milk. How many oz of fluid did the patient receive?

    A. 13 oz
    B. 24 oz
    C. 13.3 oz
    D. 13.5 oz

57. The West Wing unit has 40 patients. The East Wing unit has 0.6 as many patients. How many patients are in the West Wing?

    A. 24 patients
    B. 14 patients
    C. 17.5 patients
    D. 16.5 patients

58. A patient is receiving 1000 liters of I.V. fluid at 200 L/hr. Approximately how many hours for the 1000 L to infuse into the patient?

    A. 6 hours
    B. 4 hours
    C. 5 hours
    D. 7 hours

59. Of a pie, 3/4 remains. You want to divide the remaining equally between three patients. How much does each patient receive?

    A. 1/8
    B. 1/16
    C. 1/4
    D. 2/5

60. The nurse takes 7.2 minutes to administer medication to a patient. The nurse has 10 patients. How many minutes will it take the nurse to administer medication to all patients?

    A. 72 minutes
    B. 72.4 minutes
    C. 72.1 minutes
    D. 72.8 minutes

61. A new nurse took 12.6 minutes per patient to medicate his patients. After a year, he takes 5.2 minutes per patients. How many fewer minutes does the nurse require to administer medication?

    A. 6.4 minutes
    B. 7.4 minutes
    C. 7.5 minutes
    D. 7.6 minutes

62. $(-7) \times (-5) =$

63. What percent is 34 of 234?

64. $2.87 \div 0.3 =$

65. $2/9 \div 1/5 =$

66. A patient who had knee surgery was placed on a continuous passive motion (CPM) device that mechanically manipulates the patient's leg. The fully extended leg is measured as 0 degrees. The CPM device bends the knee measured as less than 0 degrees, which is a negative number. At the beginning of the week, the patient knee moved −5 degrees. At the end of the week, the patient was able to move his knee −14 degrees. What distance has the knee moved over the week?

    A. 9 degrees
    B. 19 degrees
    C. (−19 degrees)
    D. (−9 degrees)

67. $(-5) \div (-3) =$

68. A bag of normal saline contains 1000 L. The practitioner orders 125 L/hr. How many hours will it take to infuse 1000 L?

    A. 8 hours
    B. 6 hours
    C. 12 hours
    D. 4 hours

69. $x:84 = 1:42; x =$

70. The patients ate a tray of baked ziti and had 1/2 the tray left over. The next day the patients ate 1/4 of what was left. The patients ate the remaining baked ziti on the third day. How much baked ziti did patients eat on the third day?

    A. 1/5
    B. 1/8

C. 1/4

D. 1/3

71. **There are 98 patients. The nurse manager uses 1 nurse to 10 patients ratio and 1 CNA to 16 patients. Write an expression that shows the relationship between patients, nurses, CNAs, and the total number of clinical staff (nurse and CNAs) required to care for patients?**

A. $98 \times 8 \times 12$ = Total Number of Clinical Staff

B. (Number of Patients/10) + (Number of Patients/16) = Total Number of Clinical Staff

C. $98 + 8 + 12$ = Total Number of Clinical Staff

D. (Number of Patients × 10) × (Number of Patients × 16) = Total Number of Clinical Staff

72. $1/7 \times 1/4 =$

73. **A patient with liver failure underwent paracentesis for ascites. Fluid removed each day is 5 L. How many liters were removed in the past 2 days?**

A. 5 L

B. 1.3 L

C. 10 L

D. 1.5 L

74. $22 - x = (4 + 20)$

75. **Write an expression that shows the following relationship. Total time needed to administer medication for all patients on the day shift is the sum of the time spent on each medication pass. The nurse spends 10 minutes per patient administering morning medications; 7 minutes per patient administering noon medications; 5 minutes per patient administering 2 PM medications; and 2 minutes per patient during the shift administering PRN medication.**

A. (Number of Patients/10 min) + (Number of Patients/7 min) + (Number of Patients/5 min) + (Number of Patients/2 min) = Total Time to Administer Medication to All Patients on the Day Shift

B. (Number of Patients + 10 min) × (Number of Patients + 7 min) × (Number of Patients + 5 min) × (Number of Patients + 2 min) = Total Time to Administer Medication to All Patients on the Day shift

C. (Number of Patients + 10 min) + (Number of Patients + 7 min) + (Number of Patients + 5 min) + (Number of Patients + 2 min) = Total Time to Administer Medication to All Patients on the Day shift

D. (Number of Patients × 10 min) + (Number of Patients × 7 min) + (Number of Patients × 5 min) + (Number of Patients × 2 min) = Total Time to Administer Medication to All Patients on the Day Shift

76. $0.255 \div 4 =$

77. A patient who is recovering from a stroke undergoes physical therapy to help regain his ability to ambulate. The therapist measures the number of footsteps the patient takes regardless of the direction. In each of the three attempts, the patient took four steps backwards. The therapist recorded this as $(-4) \times 3 =$. How many steps did the patient take?

    A. $(-4$ steps$)$
    B. 4 steps
    C. $(-13$ steps$)$
    D. $(-12$ steps$)$

78. What percent is 252 of 313?

79. $y \times 16 = 32$

80. $4{:}x = 1{:}8; x =$

81. $17 - (-14) =$

82. The health care facility has a ratio of 1 CNA:2 nurses and a ratio of 1 nurse:8 patients. Your unit has 16 patients. How many CNAs would you schedule?

    A. 4 CNAs
    B. 3 CNAs
    C. 2 CNAs
    D. 1 CNA

83. The nurse manager wrote the following equation but forgot to label values in the equation. You are told to calculate the equation to determine the number of juice boxes that are expected to be delivered by dietary. How many boxes of juice will be delivered?

$$12 \times 6 + 8 = \text{Total boxes of juice}$$

    A. 168
    B. 80
    C. 86
    D. 68

84. The children's unit at the hospital encourages young patients to eat meals by awarding points that can be redeemed once a day for a prize. Failure to the eat meals causes the young patient to lose points. Six-year-old Bob received 10 points before lunch. He told the nurse that he ate all his lunch. The nurse award Bob 3 points bringing Bob's total to 15 points. However, the CNA told the nurse Bob did not eat all his lunch. The nurse deducted points using the following expression: $15 - (+3) =$. This states that a positive 3 points are being removed from the total points. What is the result of this expression?

A. 15

B. 20

C. 12

D. 5

85. A patient weight 98 lb. The practitioner orders a diet that will increase the patient's weight by 1.5 during the patient stay in the hospital. What is the patient's weight goal?

A. 140.5 lb

B. 140 lb

C. 147 lb

D. 151.5 lb

86. $1/8 \div 4/9 =$

87. $0.28 \times 0.17 =$

88. What percent is 75 of 89?

89. $x:60 = 1:4; x =$

90. $(7 \times 9) + (3 - 2) \times 7 =$

91. The health care facility developed a formula for determining CNA staffing levels. The expression is used to describe the relationships among the number of patients, CNA assignment, and required number of CNAs. How many CNAs are required for 20 patients and a CNA assignment of 0.5?

    Number of Patients $\times$ CNA Assignment = Required Number of CNAs

A. 10 CNAs

B. 14 CNAs

C. 15 CNAs

D. 16 CNAs

92. Refer to the expression in problem 91. If the nurse manager scheduled 5 CNAs, how many patients are on the unit?

A. 25 patients

B. 20 patients

C. 15 patients

D. 10 patients

93. The dietician uses the ratio of 2 hamburgers:1 patient. Your unit has five patients. How many hamburgers do you expect to receive?

    A. 12 hamburgers

    B. 10 hamburgers

    C. 16 hamburgers

    D. 15 hamburgers

94. $x:56 = 1:4; x =$

95. $x:34 = 1:16; x =$

96. $15 - (-18) =$

97. A patient was given range of motion exercise for her arm. Holding her arm straight in front of her is considered 0 degrees. Raising her arm is considered positive degrees and lowering her arm is considered negative degrees. She lowered her arm 5 degrees on Monday and 10 degrees on Tuesday. How many degrees in total did she move her arm?

    A. 5 degrees

    B. (−15 degrees)

    C. (−5 degrees)

    D. (−10 degrees)

98. By Friday, the patient in question 97 was able to lower her arm 32 degrees. How much movement since Monday she did?

    A. (−37 degrees)

    B. 37 degrees

    C. (−27 degrees)

    D. (−10 degrees)

99. Staffing requirements for nurses is based on the acuity of the patient. The acuity is assessed by the patient's diagnosis, which reflects the amount of time the nurse will likely spend per shift caring for the patient. For an average patient the acuity factor is 1. For an unstable patient the acuity factor is 2 and for a critically ill patient the acuity factor is 4. The acuity factor is divided into the normal 12 patient assignment per nurse to determine the number of patients per nurse is assigned. Write the expression that shows this relationship between the number of critically ill patients that will be assigned to a nurse.

    A. 4/8 = number of patients per nurse

    B. 12/4 = number of patients per nurse

    C. 2/8 = number of patients per nurse

    D. 8/2 = number of patients per nurse

100. Based on problem 99, write an equation that determines the number of nurses required to care for 32 average patients; 8 unstable patients; and 3 critically ill patients.

A. $(32 + (12/1)) + (8 + (12/2)) + (3 + (12/4)) =$ Total Number of Nurses
B. $(32/(12/1)) + (8/(12/2)) + (3/(12/4)) =$ Total Number of Nurses
C. $(32 + (12/1)) \times (8 + (12/2)) \times (3 + (12/4)) =$ Total Number of Nurses
D. $(32 \times (12/1)) \times (8 \times (12/2)) \times (3 \times (12/4)) =$ Total Number of Nurses

CORRECT ANSWERS AND RATIONALES

1. A. 1/5; Hint: Multiplication
2. B. 50 mg; Hint: 12.5 mg $\times$ 4 tablets
3. C. 1.1 miles; Hint: 8.4 miles $-$ 7.3 miles
4. A. 3/5; Hint: Subtraction
5. D. 4/6; Hint: Find the common denominator ($3 \times 2 = 6$); convert the numerator of the second fraction (3/6); then add the fractions (1/6 + 3/6)
6. D. 14.5 oz; Hint: 1.4 oz + 12.7 oz + 0.4 oz
7. A. 6 patients; Hint: 30 patients $\times$ 0.2
8. C. 6 hours; Hint: 1000 L $\div$ 166.67
9. C. 2/8; Hint: Divide 2/4 by 2/1; flip the fraction 1/2; multiply the fractions (2/4 $\times$ 1/2)
10. A. 49.5 minutes; Hint: 5.5 minutes $\times$ 9 patients
11. B. 2.4 minutes; Hint: 10.7 $-$ 8.3
12. $(-7) \times (-3) = 21$
13. What percent is 20 of 180 = 36?
14. $1.86 \div 0.6 = 3.1$
15. $4/9 \div 4/5 = 5/9$
16. D. -8 degrees; Hint: (-16 degrees) $-$ (-8 degrees) Like numbers result in a positive number.
17. $(-15) \div (-5) = 3$
18. A. 4 hours; Hint: 1000 L:x = 250 L:1 hour
19. x:64 = 1:32; x = 2
20. B. 2/9; Hint: Multiplication
21. B. (Number of Patients/8) + (Number of Patients/12) = Total Number of Clinical Staff; Hint: An expression shows a relationship.
22. $5/8 \times 1/4 = 5/32$
23. C. 8 L; Hint: (-3 L/day) $\times$ (-4 days) = 8 L (Negative signs are used to represent the past. Like signs result in a positive sign.)
24. $82 - x = (5 + 10)$
    $82 - x = (15)$
    $x = 15 + 82$
    $x = 97$

25. D. (Number of Patients × 30 min) + (Number of Patients × 20 min) + (Number of Patients × 15 min) + (Number of Patients × 2 min) = Total Time to Administer Medication to All Patients on the Day Shift
26. $0.225 \div 4 = 0.05625$
27. D. (−20 steps); Hint: Unlike signs
28. 23%
29. $y \times 8 = 16$
    $y = 16/8$
    $y = 2$
30. $3:x = 1:6; x = 18$
31. $7 - (-3) = 10$
32. D. 2 CNAs; Hint: x:32 patients = 0.5 CNA:8 patients
33. B. 42; Hint: Order of operations
34. C. 10; Hint: Unlike signs is a negative.
35. C. 141.6 lb; Hint: 118 lb × 1.2
36. $3/8 \div 4/5 = 15/32$
37. $0.33 \times 0.32 = 0.1056$
38. 33%; Hint: $(27/82) \times 100$
39. $x:30 = 1:5; x = 6$
40. $(4 \times 5) + (6 - 3) \times 2 =$
    $(20) + (3) \times 2 =$
    $23 + 6 = 29$
41. A. 5 CNAs; Hint: 25 × 0.2 = 5 CNAs
42. D. 25 patients; Hint: x × 0.2 = 5 CNAs, then x = 5/0.1
43. B. 50 hamburgers; Hint: x:25 patients = 2 hamburgers:1 patient
44. $x:36 = 1:9; x = 4$
45. $x:24 = 2:16; x = 3$
46. $9 - (-7) = 16$
47. B.(−24 degrees); Hint: (−18 degrees) + (−6 degrees) = (−24 degrees)
48. C. (−24 degrees); Hint: (−30 degrees) − (−6 degrees) = (−27 degrees)
48. B. (8/4) = number of patients per nurse; Hint: 8 patient normal assignments divided by the acuity factor of 4.
50. B. (20/(8/1)) + (16/(8/2)) + (8/(8/4)) = Total Number of Nurses; Hint: Calculations in the innermost parentheses are calculated first then perform the calculations in the outer parentheses.
51. A. 2/15; Hint: Multiplication
52. B. 78.6 mg; Hint: 26.2 mg × 3 tablets
53. C. 2.9 miles; Hint 9.2 miles − 6.3 miles
54. A. 5/8; Hint: Subtraction
55. D. 9/20; Hint: Find the common denominator; convert the numerator of the second fraction; then add the fractions.
56. D. 13.5 oz; Hint: 1.2 oz + 11.5 oz + 0.8 oz
57. A. 24 patients; Hint: 40 patients × 0.6

58. C. 5 hours; Hint: 1000 L ÷ 200
59. C. 1/4; Hint: Divide 3/4 by 3/1; flip the fraction 1/3; multiple the fractions (3/4 × 1/3)
60. A. 72 minutes; Hint: 7.2 minutes × 10 patients
61. B. 7.4 minutes; Hint: 12.6 − 5.2
62. $(-7) \times (-5) = 35$
63. 15%; Hint: 34/234
64. $2.87 \div 0.3 = 9.6$
65. $2/9 \div 1/5 = 1\ 1/9$
66. a. 9 degrees; Hint: (−14 degrees) − (−5 degrees) Like numbers result in a positive number.
67. $(-5) \div (-3) = 1.67$
68. A. 8 hours; Hint: 1000 L:x = 125 L:1 hour
69. x:84 = 1:42; x = 2
70. B. 1/8; Hint: Multiplication
71. B. (Number of Patients/10) + (Number of Patients/16) = Total Number of Clinical Staff; Hint: An expression shows a relationship.
72. $1/7 \times 1/4 = 1/28$
73. C. 10 L; Hint: (−5 L/day) × (−2 days) = 10 L (Negative signs are used to represent the past. Like signs result in a positive sign.)
74. $22 - x = (4 + 20)$
    $22 - x = (24)$
    $x = 24 + 22$
    $x = 46$
75. D. (Number of Patients × 10 min) + (Number of Patients × 7 min) + (Number of Patients × 5 min) + (Number of Patients × 2 min) = Total Time to Administer Medication to All Patients on the Day Shift
76. $0.255 \div 4 = 0.06375$
77. D. (−12 steps); Hint: Unlike signs
78. 81%; Hint: 252/313
79. $y \times 16 = 32$
    $y = 32/16$
    $y = 2$
80. 4:x = 1:8; x = 32; Hint: 4 × 8
81. $17 - (-14) = 31$
82. D. 1 can; Hint: x:16 patients = 0.5 CNA:8 patients
83. B. 80; Hint: Order of operations
84. C. 12; Hint: Unlike signs is a negative.
85. C. 147 lb; Hint: 98 lb × 1.5
86. $1/8 \div 4/9 = 41/72$
87. $0.28 \times 0.17 = 0.476$
88. 84%; Hint: 75/89
89. x:60 = 1:4; x = 15; Hint: 60/4

90. $(7 \times 9) + (3 - 2) \times 7 =$
    $(63) + (1) \times 7 =$
    $63 + 7 = 70$
91. A. 10 CNAs; Hint: $20 \times 0.5 = 10$ CNAs
92. D. 10 patients; Hint: $x \times 0.5 = 5$ CNAs, then $x = 5/0.5$
93. B. 10 hamburgers; Hint: x:5 patients = 2 hamburgers:1 patient
94. x:56 = 1:4; x = 14
95. x:34 = 1:16; x = 1.1251
96. $15 - (-18) = 33$
97. B. (−15 degrees); Hint: (−10 degrees) + (−5 degrees) = (−15 degrees)
98. C. (−27 degrees); Hint: (−32 degrees) − (−5 degrees) = (−27 degrees)
99. B. (12/4) = number of patients per nurse; Hint: 12 patient normal assignments divided by the acuity factor of 4.
100. B. (32/(8/1)) + (8/(8/2)) + (3/(8/4)) = Total Number of Nurses; Hint: Calculations in the innermost parentheses are calculated first then perform the calculations in the outer parentheses.

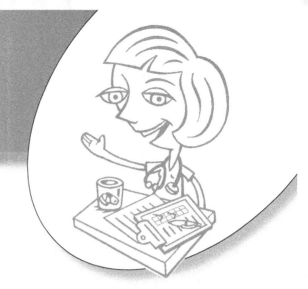

Index

Page numbers followed by *f* denote figures; those followed by *t* denote tables.